Essential Oils Guides: Box Set of Three Essential Oils Living Young Reference Manuals

By Grace Masters

Contents

Book 1

Essential Oils Guide: Reference for Living Young, Healing, Weight Loss, Aromatherapy & Recipes

By Grace Masters

Disclaimer:

This eBook is a guide for using essential oils in your daily life. It is not meant to replace any official information you have been given by your doctor. If you have any questions, you should inform your doctor, and you should discuss everything you use with your doctor when you see him or her.

RAM Internet Media, Grace Masters, and any associates are not liable for any wrong use of the oils described in this guide. This guide is for educational purposes only.

About This Guide

In this guide you will find recommendations for how to take essential oils. The following is some more information about different ways of using essential oils.

Neat: Undiluted. The essential oil is placed directly on your skin.

Diluted: The essential oil is diluted with a carrier oil like olive oil, grapeseed oil, fractionated coconut oil, and many others. Be sure you choose an all natural, high quality carrier oil for best results.

Inhale: Simply rub a drop or two of the oils between your hands, and cup them around your nose and deeply breathe in. Another way would be to put the oil on a cloth and inhale from the cloth.

Diffuse: Place 3-4 drops of the essential oil in an essential oil diffuser with distilled water.

Internal: For Therapeutic Grade essential oils, you can take them internally. Either, place a drop under your tongue, combine a drop with water, milk, or juice, or place them in a vegetable capsule along with a carrier oil and swallow. Some essential oils are also good to cook with.

I hope you enjoy the information contained within this guide and find good health using high quality essential oils. They can be life changing.

What are Essential Oils?

Many of us have used essential oils in one form or another – in scented bath salts, in aromatic candles, in soaps, in food, in potpourri, in cosmetics, and a whole lot of other products. We may not, however, know what essential oils really are. These oils have fragrance, certainly, and come in a variety of scents. These have many physical and mental benefits. This guide explains the basics of essential oils, describes many of the most common oils and how to use the, and gives small recipes for using the essential oils in your household, for your pet, and for your health.

Essential oils are oils extracted from certain fragrant plants and herbs like rose, rosemary, lavender, peppermint, licorice, anise, lemon, lemongrass, etc. They are highly volatile and easily spread their fragrance in air, which is why they are used to produce a number of aromatic products. The name "essential" comes from the word "essence." It was once thought that essential oils represented the very essence of flavor and odor. So, they are "essential" solely for that reason. They can offer some quick fixes for your body and mind.

How Do We Get Essential Oils?

There are several methods of extracting essential oil from plants. These include:

- Distillation, which is the most common method of applying steam or water and steam to plant material in a sealed sill and removing the volatile components of the plant.
- Enfleurage, which is a process of embedding the flower petals or fragrant herbs in purified and odorless fat and letting the essential oils infuse the fat; the fat is then washed with alcohol to separate the oils.

- Maceration, in which the flowers are soaked in hot oil that absorbs the essence; the essential oil is then decanted out.
- Solvent extracted methods, which use other chemical solvents to extract oils from plants that have low yield.
- And other processes like mechanical pressing.

Can All Plants Produce Essential Oils?

Only a thousand or so plants out of the hundreds of thousands of known plant species are recognized as being able to give us essential oils.

Plants store the oils in the form of micro droplets (microscopic droplets you can't see) in certain glands. The oils then diffuse through the glandular walls and spread over the plant's surface, before evaporating and filling the air with fragrance.

Oils can be extracted from flowers, leaves, roots, and wood. It is not very clear why plants need essential oils, but it may be to attract insects to flowers or protect the plants from parasites and animals.

How Long Have Essential Oils Been Used?

Essential oils have been used for quite a long time. Archeological evidence shows that distillation of plants to prepare distilled aromatic waters or floral waters has been done since the Middle Ages. Even further back we had Zosimus of Panoplis, a fifth century writer, writing about what he called "divine water." The first known records of essential oil use are from ancient civilizations of Persia, India, and Egypt. There is also evidence that essential oils were extracted with some simple methods in ancient Rome, Greece, and the Orient.

Originally, the plant materials were simply infused in oil, left in a bottle in the sun and then the aromatic oil was poured out for use. More often, the plants and their resins were used directly. Then the Arabs brought their crude distillation methods, having already distilled ethyl alcohol from sugar. With their knowledge, alcohol could now be used as the new solvent for essential oil distillation. Purer oil could be extracted from plants.

What Essential Oils Were Used in the Past?

The method of distillation that the Arabs established slowly spread to Europe in the Middle Ages. Medieval pharmacies listed oils of rosemary, rose, calamus, cedarwood, costus, turpentine, spike, sage, myrrh, benzoin, and cinnamon. Alchemist Paracelsus played a big role in urging physicians to extract oils from the leaves, flowers, roots and wood of plants. In the Middle Ages, floral waters were used as digestive tonics, in perfumes, for trading and in cooking.

With trade and travel across the Silk Route, other spices were introduced from India, China and what is Southeast Asia today, by Marco Polo and other travelers from his time. Nutmeg, cardamom, and other spices were soon turned into essential oils. By the mid-eighteenth century, Europe knew about hundred essential oils. Slowly their chemical natures began to be understood and better methods of mass production were invented in the late 1800s and early 1900s.

The young United States already knew about peppermint and turpentine oils before 1800. Over the next few decades, oils of wintergreen, sassafras, sweet birch, and wormwood became the most commercially popular of all the known essential oils in the country.

What Are Essential Oils Good For?

High quality essential oils have been found to provide several benefits for a long time. First of all, they offer pure pleasure and emotional benefits. Anyone who loves a sniff of fragrant flowers or kitchen spices will recognize that. They are not only fragrant, but also therapeutic. Each oil has its own healing profile.

There are other benefits for which we buy essential oils. They are known to relieve stress, soothe you into sleep, energize you, or even lift a depression. They can ease aches and pain, as pungent eastern liniments can do, or treat a wide range of emotional and physical problems.

When buying essential oils, it is useful to know what each essential oil is recommended for. You can then begin to enjoy the benefits that these oils have been providing for over 5000 years.

Precautions

- Essential oils are highly concentrated and must never be taken internally unless you buy the 100% pure Therapeutic Grade brands of essential oils, which include Young Living, Doterra, Rocky Mountain, and others.
- Some people can have allergic reaction to these oils, so you should test your skin first to see if yours is sensitive to a particular oil.
- These oils should never be applied undiluted on babies or very young children because they could make the skin burn.
- Many oils can be stored for years without losing their aroma, though some may need to be stored refrigerated.
- Oils should always be kept in sealed dark bottles away from direct sunlight, and preferably in a cool place.
- When pregnant, avoid the following essential oils: Aniseed, cedarwood, chamomile, cinnamon, clary sage, clove, ginger, jasmine, lemon, nutmeg, rosemary, and sage. During the first trimester, you may want to avoid all essential oils. Discuss their use with your doctor.
- Be sure to store your essential oils in a dark, cool place for maximum lifespan. If they are stored correctly, a bottle of an essential oil could last from 5 to 10 years.

Why Use Essential Oils

Essential oils can help you achieve better health without all the toxic chemicals present in most households today. In fact, using them regularly is an ideal way tow enhance your health as well as heal some of the common ailments that may be prevalent in your home. Depending on the type of oil used, there are a wide range of benefits. These oils have been around for many years commonly for cosmetic, health, emotional, and spiritual purposes and millions of people continue to use them as they have been used over thousands of years.

Essential oils are non-toxic. They are easy to use and are made from natural extracts, which are extracted under stringent conditions to ensure quality. These natural products also react effectively with the body to and do not provide unwanted and sometimes dangerous side effects of traditional medication. The oils are tailored for ease of use. In fact, you can add them to baths, apply to your body, and use them the surfaces within your, or diffuse them to enhance your home's fragrance while providing effective aromatherapy.

There are many great reasons to use essential oils. Just a few of the positive benefits of using essential oils are described in the following paragraphs.

Inspiring Positive Emotions

The brain is the key body part that has control of the rest of the body. When you use essential oils, they can have a positive effect on your brain. Because the brain is the center of emotions and memory, the oils may trigger the brain in a positive manner when these oils are inhaled or diffused.

This positive reaction in the brain is one of the reasons people love to use essential oils for aromatherapy. To achieve this there is a range of oil products, which are used for diffusion, bathing, massage, or topical application depending on the reason you are using the oil.

The use of the oils can reduce the effects of insomnia and help promote sleep by increasing relaxation and decreasing anxiety. When sprinkled on the pillow before bedtime, the oils are known to induce a restful sleep. Some calming oils include lavender, orange, peppermint, and Jasmine.

Improving Physical Fitness and Health

Essential oils can positively impact both physical fitness and health. These oils can help detoxify the body to remove any harmful and excessive substances within the body.

In this regard, using essential oils and supplement infused essential oils provides an effective way to clean the body, manage body weight, and improve performance of body metabolic systems. Rubbing an oil like peppermint on your stomach can help to relieve the stomach of digestive upsets and also to relieve heartburn, gas, and irritable bowel diseases among others. Using essential oil products can also help prevent you from contracting bacteria, viral and fungal infections. This includes some bacteria that are resistant to antibiotics and penicillin. If you are already sick, chances are, an essential oil can help you get over the illness in an effective way without the risk of unwanted side effects that traditional pharmaceuticals carry.

Enhancing Skin

The skin is the body's largest organ. Among other factors, it offers protection for the body, and it is vitally important to your overall health. For this reason it requires special care. Because it covers your body, skin is exposed to harmful chemicals, radiation, and dirt, which makes it even more important to keep your skin as healthy as possible. Using essential oils has become popular part of many skin care regimens.

Essential oils can skin cell growth as well promote a healthy skin complexion making it look young and healthy. The oils also promote softening of the skin ensuring it performs effectively as the body's largest organ. Common essential oil products for skin include lavender oil and frankincense.

Common Essential Oils and Their Uses

While there are over 1000 essential oils, the follow section details several of the most common and popular essential oils.

Angelica root

- **Physical:** Dull skin, gout, psoriasis, toxin build-up, and water retention.
- **Emotional:** Exhaustion, nervousness, and stress.
- **Caution:** Avoid when Pregnant. Phototoxic, so take care in sunlight after application.

Anise

- **Physical:** Bronchitis, colds, coughs, flatulence, flu, muscle aches, and rheumatism.
- **Emotional:** Depression.
- **How to use:** Inhale or diffuse in the morning as a pick-me-up.

Basil

- **Physical:** Bronchitis, colds, coughs, exhaustion, flatulence, flu, gout, insect bites, insect repellent, muscle aches, rheumatism, and sinusitis.
- **Emotional:** Fatigue, exhaustion, burnout, memory and concentration, anxiety, fear, and nervousness.

- **How to use:** Apply topically either neat (oil directly on skin) or with carrier oil like coconut oil (1 drop per 1-3 tablespoons of carrier). If your Basil oil is high quality, you may add it to cooking as well.

Bay laurel

- **Physical:** Amenorrhea, colds, flu, loss of appetite, tonsillitis, bronchitis, and rheumatoid arthritis.
- **Emotional:** Confidence and mental confusion.
- **How to use:** Dilute 1 drop with 1 drop of a carrier oil. Apply several drops (2-4) on location, apply to chakras and vitaflex points, inhale, or diffuse.

Benzoin

- **Physical:** Arthritis, bronchitis, chapped skin, coughing, and laryngitis. This oil has antiseptic properties.
- **Emotional:** Insecurity.
- **How to use:** Use undiluted an apply directly to area or vitaflex points. Inhale or diffuse.

Bergamot

- **Physical:** Acne, abscesses, anxiety, boils, cold sores, cystitis, halitosis, itching, loss of appetite, oily skin, and psoriasis.
- **Emotional:** Anger, anxiety, confidence, depression, stress, fatigue, fear, peace, happiness, insecurity, and loneliness.
- **How to use:** Apply topically either neat (oil directly on skin) or with carrier oil like coconut oil (1 drop per 1-3

tablespoons of carrier). It can also be used in cooking or in non-acidic beverages if you have a high quality brand.

Note: *Bergamot is citrus oil, and it may cause issues if the area you apply it to is exposed to the sun within 24 hours. All citrus oils have this photosensitivity issue, so be aware.*

Bois de rose (Rosewood)

- **Physical:** Acne, colds, dry skin, dull skin, fever, flu, frigidity, headache, oily skin, scars, sensitive skin, stress, and stretch marks.
- **Emotional:** Depression and emotional imbalance.

Cajeput

- **Physical:** Asthma, bronchitis, coughs, muscle aches, oily skin, rheumatism, sinusitis, sore throat, and spots.
- **Emotional:** Fatigue and mental confusion.

Cardamom

- **Physical:** Appetite loss of, colic, and halitosis.
- **Emotional:** Fatigue, stress, shame, and guilt.
- **How to use:** Dilute 1 drop with 1 drop of a carrier oil. Apply several drops (2-4) on location, apply to chakras and vitaflex points, inhale, or diffuse.

Carrot seed

- **Physical:** Eczema, gout, mature skin, toxin build-up, water retention.
- **Emotional:** Anxiety, confusion, exhaustion, mood swings and stress.
- **How to use:** Dilute 1 drop with 1 drop of a carrier oil. Apply several drops (2-4) on location, apply to chakras and vitaflex points, inhale, or diffuse.

Cedarwood Atlas

- **Physical:** Acne, arthritis, bronchitis, coughing, cystitis, dandruff, and dermatitis.
- **Emotional:** Anxiety, fear, insecurity, and stress.

Cedarwood

- **Physical:** Acne, arthritis, bronchitis, coughs, cystitis, dandruff, dermatitis, insect repellent, and stress.
- **Emotional:** Anxiety, fear and insecurity, calming.
- **How to use:** Apply topically either neat (oil directly on skin) or with carrier oil like coconut oil (1 drop per 1-3 tablespoons of carrier).

German Chamomile

- **Physical:** Abscesses, allergies, arthritis, boils, colic, cuts, cystitis, dermatitis, dysmenorrhea, earache, flatulence, hair,

headache, inflamed skin, insect bites, insomnia, nausea, neuralgia, rheumatism, sores, sprains, strains, wounds.
- **Emotional:** Anger, anxiety, depression, fear, irritability, loneliness, PMS, and stress.
- **How to use:** Apply topically either neat (oil directly on skin) or with carrier oil like coconut oil (1 drop per 1-3 tablespoons of carrier).

Roman Chamomile

- **Physical:** Abscesses, allergies, arthritis, boils, colic, cuts, cystitis, dermatitis, dysmenorrhea, earache, flatulence, hair, headache, inflamed skin, insect bites, nausea, neuralgia, PMS, rheumatism, sores, sprains, strains, and wounds, and bee stings.
- **Emotional:** Anger, anxiety, depression, fear, irritability, loneliness, insomnia, stress, and purposelessness.
- **How to use:** Apply topically either neat (oil directly on skin) or with carrier oil like coconut oil (1 drop per 1-3 tablespoons of carrier). It can also be used in cooking or in non-acidic, non-dairy beverages if you have a high quality brand.

Note: *If you have sensitive skin, do a patch test first.*

Cinnamon

- **Physical:** Constipation, exhaustion, flatulence, lice, low blood pressure, rheumatism, scabies.
- **Emotional:** Concentration, emotional and mental fatigue, healthy relationships, and healthy sexuality.

- **How to use:** Apply topically diluted with carrier oil like coconut oil in a minimum of a 1 to 3 ratio. It can also be used in cooking or in non-acidic, non-dairy beverages if you have a high quality brand.

Citronella

- **Physical:** Excessive perspiration, fatigue, headache, insect repellent, and oily skin.
- **Emotional:** Mind fog and tension.
- **How to use:** Dilute 1 drop with 1 drop of a carrier oil. Apply several drops (2-4) on location, apply to chakras and vitaflex points, inhale, or diffuse.

Clary Sage

- **Physical:** Amenorrhea, asthma, coughing, gas, labor pains, hormone balancing, heavy periods, cramps, and sore throat.
- **Emotional:** Anxiety, fatigue, exhaustion, fear, loneliness, stress, and clarity.
- **How to use:** Apply topically either neat (oil directly on skin) or with carrier oil like coconut oil (1 drop per 1-3 tablespoons of carrier). It can also be used in cooking or in non-acidic, non-dairy beverages if you have a high quality brand.

Clove

- **Physical:** Arthritis, asthma, bronchitis, immune system, rheumatism, sprains, toothache, and digestive support.

- **Emotional:** Memory and concentration, fatigue, depression, breaking victimization patterns, and healthy boundaries.
- **How to use:** Apply topically diluted with carrier oil like coconut oil in a minimum of a 1 to 3 ratio. It can also be used in cooking or in non-acidic, non-dairy beverages if you have a high quality brand.

Coriander

- **Physical:** Aches, arthritis, colic, gout, indigestion, nausea, and rheumatism.
- **Emotional:** Fatigue and irritation.
- **How to use:** Dilute 1 drop with 1 drop of a carrier oil. Apply several drops (2-4) on location, apply to chakras and vitaflex points, inhale, or diffuse.

Cypress

- **Physical:** Excessive perspiration, hemorrhoids, oily skin, rheumatism, and varicose veins.
- **Emotional:** Confidence, grief, memory, and concentration.

Elemi

- **Physical:** Bronchitis, catarrh, extreme coughing, mature skin, scars, stress, and wounds.
- **Emotional:** Agitation and grief.

Eucalyptus Globulous

- **Physical:** Arthritis, bronchitis, catarrh, cold sores, colds, coughing, fever, flu, poor circulation, and sinusitis.
- **Emotional:** Concentration and memory.

Fennel

- **Physical:** Bruises, cellulite, flatulence, gums, halitosis, mouth, nausea, obesity, toxin build-up, and water retention.
- **Emotional:** Fatigue and emotional imbalance.

Frankincense

- **Physical:** Anxiety, asthma, bronchitis, extreme coughing, scars, and stretch marks.
- **Emotional:** Anxiety, depression, fatigue exhaustion and burnout, fear, grief, happiness and peace, insecurity, loneliness, panic and panic attacks, and stress.
- **How to use:** Dilute 1 drop with 1 drop of a carrier oil. Apply several drops (2-4) on location, apply to chakras and vitaflex points, inhale, or diffuse.

Galbanum

- **Physical:** Immune system abscesses, acne, boils, bronchitis, cuts, lice, mature skin, muscle aches, poor circulation, rheumatism, scars, sores, stretch marks, and wounds.
- **Emotional:** Emotional rigidity, mood swings, nervousness, and stress.

Geranium

- **Physical:** Acne, cellulite, dull skin, lice, menopause, and oily skin.
- **Emotional:** Anxiety, depression, happiness, mood imbalance, and stress.

Ginger

- **Physical:** Aching muscles, arthritis, nausea, and poor circulation.
- **Emotional:** Fatigue exhaustion and burnout.
- **How to use:** Dilute 1 drop with 1 drop of a carrier oil. Apply several drops (2-4) on location, apply to chakras and vitaflex points, inhale, or diffuse.

Grapefruit

- **Physical:** Cellulite, dull skin, toxin build-up, and water retention.
- **Emotional:** Confidence, fear depression, happiness and peace, and stress.

Helichrysum

- **Physical:** Abscesses, acne, boils, burns, cuts, dermatitis, eczema, irritated skin, and wounds.
- **Emotional:** Grief, loneliness, panic and panic attacks, and shock.

Hyssop

- **Physical:** Bruises, coughing, sore throat, and respiratory system.
- **Emotional:** Concentration and nervousness.

Jasmine

- **Physical:** Dry skin, labor pains, and sensitive skin.
- **Emotional:** Stress, depression, fear, fatigue exhaustion and burnout, confidence, and anger.
- **How to use:** Apply several drops (2-4) directly on location, apply to chakras and vitaflex points, inhale, or diffuse.

Juniper berry

- **Physical:** Cellulite, gout, hemorrhoids, obesity, rheumatism, toxin build-up, and urinary system.
- **Emotional:** Agitation and negative energy.

Lavender

- **Physical:** Acne, allergies, anxiety, asthma, athlete's foot, bruises, burns, chicken pox, colic, cuts, cystitis, depression, dermatitis, earache, flatulence, headache, hypertension, insect bites, insect repellent, itching, labor pains, migraine, oily skin, rheumatism, scabies, scars, sores, sprains, strains, stress, stretch marks, vertigo, and whooping cough.
- **Emotional:** Anxiety, depression, irritability, panic attacks, and stress. Promotes honest communication.

- **How to use:** Lavender is known as a universal oil, and there are many ways to use it. Diffuse or inhale directly. Apply topically either neat (oil directly on skin) or with carrier oil like coconut oil (1 drop per 1-3 tablespoons of carrier). It can also be used in cooking or in non-acidic beverages if you have a high quality brand.

F

Lemon

- **Physical:** Athlete's foot, colds, corns, dull skin, flu, oily skin, spots, varicose veins, and warts.
- **Emotional:** Fear, happiness, and peace; memory, and concentration.

Lemongrass

- **Physical:** Acne, athlete's foot, digestion, excessive perspiration, flatulence, insect repellent, muscle aches, oily skin, scabies, and stress. This oil is also an insect repellant.
- **Emotional:** Fatigue and mental confusion.

Linden blossom

- **Physical:** Headache, migraine, Acne, dull skin, oily skin, scars, spots, and wrinkles.
- **Emotional:** Insomnia, stress, and tension.

Marjoram

- **Physical:** Aching muscles, arthritis, cramps, migraine, neuralgia, rheumatism, spasm, and sprains.
- **Emotional:** Mood swings, PMS symptoms, and stress.

Melaleuca (Tea Tree)

- **Physical:** Treating wounds, yeast, acne, cold sores, and cleaning.
- **Emotional:** Promotes healthy boundaries, helps with codependency, and helps with saying no.
- **How to use:** Diffuse or inhale directly. Apply topically either neat (oil directly on skin) or with carrier oil like coconut oil (1 drop per 1-3 tablespoons of carrier).

Melissa

- **Physical:** Flu, indigestion, herpes, nausea, shingles, and cold sores.
- **Emotional:** Agitation, anxiety, dementia, and nervous tension.
- **How to use:** Apply several drops (2-4) directly on location, apply to chakras and vitaflex points, inhale, or diffuse.

Myrrh

- **Physical:** Amenorrhea, athlete's foot, bronchitis, chapped skin, gums, halitosis, itching, and ringworm.
- **Emotional:** Emotional imbalance and creativity.

- **How to use:** Apply several drops (2-4) directly on location, apply to chakras and vitaflex points, inhale, or diffuse.

Myrtle

- **Physical:** Acne, asthma, coughs, hemorrhoids, and irritated skin.
- **Emotional:** Addiction and self-destructive behavior and depression.

Neroli

- **Physical:** Mature skin, oily skin, scars, and stretch marks.
- **Emotional:** Anxiety, depression, anger, irritability, panic attacks, and stress.

Niaouli

- **Physical:** Acne, bronchitis, colds, coughs, dull skin, oily skin, sore throat, and whooping cough.
- **Emotional:** Concentration and mental fog.

Nutmeg

- **Physical:** Arthritis, constipation, muscle aches, nausea, neuralgia, poor circulation, rheumatism, and slow digestion.
- **Emotional:** Mental fatigue.

Bitter orange

- **Physical:** Colds, constipation, dull skin, flatulence, flu, gums, mouth, and slow digestion.
- **Emotional:** Anger, confidence, depression, fear, happiness, peace, and stress.

Oregano

- **Physical:** Coughs, digestion, respiration, pain, inflammation. It is an antibacterial, antiviral, antifungal, and antiparasitic.
- **Emotional:** Insecurity.
- **How to use:** Dilute with a carrier oil in a 4 to 1 ratio for external use. Adults may add up to 10 drops daily in a juice, milk, or water. Do not use heavily for more than 2 weeks at a time.

Parsley

- **Physical:** Congestion, digestion, diuretic, immune system, kidney infections and stones.
- **Emotional:** Frigidity.

Patchouli

- **Physical:** Acne, cellulite, chapped skin, dandruff, dermatitis, eczema, mature skin, and oily skin.
- **Emotional:** Fatigue, frigidity exhaustion, and stress.

Black pepper

- **Physical:** Aching muscles, arthritis, detox, constipation, muscle cramps, poor circulation, and sluggish digestion.
- **Emotional:** Anxiety, fatigue, and concentration.

Peppermint

- **Physical:** Asthma, colic, exhaustion, fever, flatulence, headache, nausea, scabies, sinusitis, and vertigo.
- **Emotional:** Fatigue, exhaustion, and burnout. It also helps memory and concentration.
- **How to use:** Dilute with a carrier oil and rub on temples. Rub a drop on your stomach for a stomachache. Also, inhale for quick relief.

Petitgrain

- **Physical:** Rapid heartbeat and insomnia.
- **Emotional:** Anxiety and panic.

Pine

- **Physical:** Colds, congestion, cough, flu, lungs, and sinusitis.
- **Emotional:** Depression, fatigue, and nervous exhaustion.

Rose

- **Physical:** Eczema, mature skin.

- **Emotional:** Anger, anxiety, frigidity, depression grief, menopause, happiness and peace, loneliness, panic, panic attacks, and stress.

Rosemary

- **Physical:** Aching muscles, arthritis, dandruff, dull skin, exhaustion, gout, hair care, muscle cramping, neuralgia, poor circulation, rheumatism, immune system, and respiratory problems.
- **Emotional:** Fatigue, exhaustion, and burnout; confidence, memory and concentration.

Sandalwood

- **Physical:** Bronchitis, chapped and dry skin, laryngitis, oily skin, strep throat, urinary tract problems.
- **Emotional:** Anxiety, depression, exhaustion and burnout, fear, grief, irritability, and stress.

Spearmint

- **Physical:** Asthma, exhaustion, flatulence, headache, nausea, and scabies.
- **Emotional:** Depression and mental fatigue.

Thyme

- **Physical:** Arthritis, bronchitis, candida, cuts, dermatitis, gastritis, and laryngitis.

- **Emotional:** Concentration and memory.

Vetiver

- **Physical:** Acne, arthritis, muscular aches, oily skin, and rheumatism.
- **Emotional:** Anger, anxiety, exhaustion, insomnia, fear, grief, insecurity, and stress.

Violet leaf

- **Physical:** Bronchitis, insomnia, liver congestion, sluggish circulation, and problem skin.
- **Emotional:** Fear, nostalgia, obsession, and shyness.

White Fir

- **Physical:** Pain, respiratory system, muscle, and bone.
- **Emotional:** Addiction, abuse, anger, and co-dependency.
- **How to use:** Diffuse or inhale directly. Apply topically either neat (oil directly on skin) or with carrier oil like coconut oil (1 drop per 1-3 tablespoons of carrier).

Yarrow

- **Physical:** Acne, arthritis, inflammation, hair care, hypertension, and insomnia.
- **Emotional:** Insomnia, stress, and tension.

Ylang Ylang

- **Physical:** Hypertension, menopause and PMS symptoms, and palpitations.
- **Emotional:** Anger, depression, frigidity, mood swings, PMS, and stress. It releases negative emotions such as anger, possessiveness or low self-esteem and nourishes positive emotions such as confidence, self-love, and spiritual awareness.
- **How to use:** Apply several drops (2-4) on affected location, apply to chakras/vitaflex points, directly inhale or diffuse. It can be used as a dietary supplement as well.

Common Ailments and Essential Oil Treatment

The use of essential oils to treat illness pretty common, especially after science has proven that they do work with basic health problems. The good news is that essential oils are usually safer to use than drugs.

Like medications, however, you can't just swap one essential oil for another. Knowing exactly what type to use for a specific ailment is crucial if you want it to work. In here, you will find a list of some of the most common ailments and what oils can be used to treat them.

Note: *This information is not intended to cure any disease or illness. Please use knowledge of your own body and situation before using essential oils for illness. If you have any question as to whether or not an oil is safe for you, please discuss it with your doctor.*

Aching Muscles

There are several oils you can use for muscle pain including basil, cypress, rosemary, roman chamomile, lavender, elemi, wintergreen, clary sage, and marjoram.

A 1% solution of these oils can be massaged directly on the aching muscles at least once a day. If you suffer from chronic pain, however, a 5% solution would be best. If a massage is not to your liking, you can try mixing the oil with cold water and using it as a cold compress.

Acne

Tea tree oil is the one most commonly used essential oils for acne. You can apply it directly on the pimple and achieve an overnight fix. Tea tree oil can be quite harsh though, especially if you have sensitive skin. A good replacement would be lavender and rosemary, both applied the same way if you find that your skin does not handle tea tree oil.

ADHD

A study published in the American Medical Association reveals that the use of essential oils on patients with ADD/ADHD helps increase their focus and concentration. Headed by Dr. Terry Friedman, the oils were simply inhaled by the patients to produce results. These oils were cedarwood, lavender, and vetiver. You might also try diffusing these oils to see if you get results.

Allergies

Seasonal allergies can be treated with lavender, lemon, or peppermint. Contrary to popular belief, you don't have to smell them but rather, apply them on the bottom of your feet. Cover your foot with a sock to get better results.

Arthritis

Oils that work for arthritis-caused pain includes: rosemary, lavender, peppermint, marjoram, and eucalyptus. All of these can be applied directly on the aching joints if your skin is not too sensitive to the oils' full strengths.

Asthma

Asthma responds well to peppermint, rosemary, ginger, geranium, eucalyptus, and frankincense. The ones mentioned typically work best when used in-between attacks. Simply rub them on the chest area to prevent tightening of the lungs. To treat attacks as they occur, lavender can be used as steam.

Bronchitis

Bronchitis can be treated with lavender, myrtle, rosemary, pine needle, and cedar wood. Use it as a steam, dropping around 4 drops of the oil in hot water and slowly inhaling the steam.

Bruises

Bruises respond best to lavender, cypress, geranium, lemon grass, and helichrysum. You can apply them directly to the wound to relieve pain and restore blood flow.

Burns

Burns are best addressed immediately using lavender, Melrose, roman chamomile, and rose oils. You can apply them directly on first-degree burns. Second and third degree burns are best addressed medically.

Colds

Lemon oil is best used for the cold. You can rub them directly on your lymph nodes located a few centimeters below the ears.

Cold Sores

You can apply lavender, tea tree oil, and eucalyptus to cold sores. Note though that it is usually best to dilute these first with grape seed oil or another carrier oil before application.

Congestion

Eucalyptus works well with congestion problems, typically inhaled in steam form. You can also use a combination of rosemary, eucalyptus, and lemon as a rubbing agent on the nose, chest, and forehead.

Constipation

Massaging oils on the stomach works well but for best results, try drinking a combination of olive oil and lemon oil on an empty stomach in the morning. Ratio should be 1 is to 1.

Cough

For coughs, try combining one drop of each ingredient and drinking them: lemon oil, frankincense oil, orange oil, peppermint oil, and honey as needed.

Cuts

Thyme, thieves, and tea tree oil all work well when applied directly on the wound 3 times a day. It's best to dilute them with a carrier oil before application. Infected wounds work better with clive while bleeding wounds respond to geranium.

Diarrhea

For diarrhea, you can use thyme, peppermint, eucalyptus, and chamomile. Simply combine 6 drops of any of the oils with 1 teaspoon of carrier oil and massage it on the stomach. You can also use a combination of frankincense and carrier oil taken 3 times a day.

Eczema

This skin problem is best treated with lavender oil mixed with carrier oil and applied directly on the skin. If you are allergic to lavender, you can use thyme or geranium.

Fever

The mix usually changes depending on the age of the child but for a 12-year old, you can combine 5 drops pine, 3 drops eucalyptus, and 2 drops frankincense. Add some carrier oil and put the whole mix in warm bath water where the child can wash.

Flu

Use frankincense oil, rubbing a single drop on the chest area to help relive flu symptoms.

Headache

Fix a pounding headache or migraine by putting a few drops of ginger or lavender in water – preferably 15 degrees Fahrenheit. Soak your hand in it for a few minutes. Alternatively, rub a few drops of peppermint on your temples and over your forehead.

Hypertension

The best oils for hypertension include ylang-ylang, lavender, and sweet marjoram. You can massage them on the skin or inhale their relaxing scent to help decrease blood pressure.

Insect Bites

Use peppermint, basil, thyme, Melrose, lavender, or tea tree oil for insect bites. Apply a diluted version directly on the skin.

Kidney Infection

For kidney problems, you can choose between fennel, German chamomile, and juniper. Ingestion is the best way to use them, so it's best to make them into a pill form by putting drops of the oils into a vegetable pill shell. If not, you can still use the oil by applying them on the skin, directly on top of the kidney.

Laryngitis

Lavender, tea tree, and eucalyptus oils all work against laryngitis. Inhale them to get the best results.

Menopause

Menopause is inevitable but with the right oils, it can be a more comfortable process. Use chamomile for emotional symptoms, lavender to boost estrogen, and peppermint for hot flashes. These can all be taken as part of aromatherapy.

Migraine

You can cure migraine using the same technique as with headaches. You can also use lavender, eucalyptus, roman chamomile, and spearmint for the problem. Simply combine around 8 drops of the oil with 1 ounce of carrier oil and massage the mix on your temples.

Nausea

Put lavender or peppermint in a tissue or a handkerchief and simply smell the aroma whenever nausea strikes. Alternatively, rub a drop of peppermint oil in a circle around your belly button.

PMS

For PMS, lavender is usually gentle enough to be rubbed directly on the skin. You can also inhale it as is. If you prefer aromatherapy methods, the best oils to use would be geranium, jasmine, rose, clary sage, and chamomile.

Sores

Infected sores are best treated with oregano, Melrose, tea tree oil, and thyme. Dilute them first using carrier oil and then use around 3 drops directly on the skin.

Sore Throat

For sore throat, you can use the same system as with laryngitis. If you want something quick and easy, add around 3 drops of peppermint in tea and get that menthol relief for the sore throat.

Upset Stomach

Upset stomachs can be fixed with peppermint oil. Just rub a drop of the oil around the belly button and wait for a few minutes. You can also rub the oil on the feet and put on socks to help the body with the absorption. You can also try using techniques for nausea and constipation.

Remember, it's usually a good idea to dilute essential oils before ingesting them or applying them topically. Dilution is best done by combining carrier oil like vegetable oil, olive oil, coconut oil, or another favorite carrier with the natural oils. If you're going to inhale or diffuse the oil however, diluting them is not necessary.

Essential Oils for Weight Loss

Little did you know, aside from undergoing the knife or using supplements to aid in weight loss, you could also try essential oils, such as peppermint, grapefruit, bergamot, sandalwood, and the list goes on. These essential oils could have a positive impact in your weight loss endeavors if combined with a healthy diet and exercise.

Nonetheless, there's no full guarantee that these oils could dramatically make your waist smaller, but they could have a positive impact on your mood and increase your body's energy and vitality. The following are some of the most effective essential oils for weight management and weight loss.

Peppermint

Peppermint is the perfect essential oil that could treat your upset stomach and promote better digestion. As a matter of fact, according to Dr. Alan Hirsch, peppermint oil could be attributed to weight loss because it works on the brain's satiety center and gives the feeling of a full stomach for a longer period.

Directions: Before meals, just add a few drops of peppermint oil to a handkerchief and inhale it; this would curb your appetite. Also, you could add a drop or two to a glass of water and drink it before meals.

Grapefruit

One of the main ingredients of grapefruit oil is the limonene. This substance triggers the body to release fatty acids into the bloodstream and converts them into usable energy. That's why grapefruit essential oil could reduce water retention and effectively dissolve fat.

Directions: Grapefruit essential oil could efficiently control your appetite, because it is an appetite suppressant. Just inhale a few drops of it whenever you're feeling hungry or craving for something.

Bergamot

One of the causes of obesity is emotional stress. Fortunately, bergamot oil could fight this feeling, eliminating the possibilities of overeating. It works in a way where the endocrine system is stimulated and the essential oil provides a sense of wellbeing and calmness, while lowering stress at the same time.

Directions: You could add lavender essential oil to bergamot oil and it'll enhance the effects dramatically. Additionally, just like your peppermint oil, all you need to do is add a drop of it on your handkerchief and inhale it before having a meal. Aside from curbing your appetite, it could also make you feel more relaxed.

Sandalwood

Sandalwood promotes the feeling of wellbeing. Likewise, it's also quite popular because of the medicinal properties it has, such as being an astringent, skin treatment, and sedative. Though, known to be the most important function of sandalwood is that it has the capability of altering the negative cell programming, as well as the behavior. Therefore, it has been noted that sandalwood could have an effect on the brain's ability to resist temptation, resulting to self-control and appetite control.

Directions: Just inhale sandalwood before meals to experience its effects.

Tangerine

Tangerine essential oil is a citrus-based oil that could assist you in your weight loss goals. Most people use this oil as a skin toner, for it helps in reducing the appearance of stretch marks, cellulite, and scars. Likewise, tangerine oil could also promote feelings of happiness, reduce anxiety, and regulate the metabolism. Keep in mind though, it's not advisable to go out in the sun after applying tangerine.

Directions: Combine tangerine essential oil with bergamot or lavender oil to experience optimum results.

Rose Geranium

This essential oil is best known for its mood lifting properties. Furthermore, experts suggest that the properties of rose geranium essential oil could reduce the appearance of cellulite, as well as the effects of fluid retention or edema, resulting to well balanced hormones. Other health benefits of rose geranium are, anti-fungal, toxin flusher, anti-parasite, and skin care agent. When taking this oil, no need to worry about any harmful effects, because it has a GRAS rating from the FDA, which means it's safe for consumption.

Sweet Orange

It's ideal to help the body have a better circulation and increase the rate of metabolism, resulting in faster weight loss.

Sweet Fennel

Considered to be an appetite suppressant that could aid in weight loss, increase metabolism, dispel gas, balance hormones, and promotes better digestion.

Lemon Oil

Lemon essential oil is extracted from the rind of the fruit, and one of its properties is that it could boost the metabolism, which dissolves fat faster and removes the toxins from the body. No need to undergo liposuction with the help of lemon oil.

Directions: Just apply lemon essential oil on the skin and notice how it dissolves those extra fat and cellulite. Likewise, it could also be used internally to make it more effective.

For internal use, just add a drop of it in a glass of water and drink throughout the day to detoxify the body.

On the other hand, by mixing 3-4 drops of lemon oil with 1 tsp. coconut oil, you could come up with a solution that you could apply all over your belly, buttocks, and hips to tighten the skin.

Ocotea Oil

This essential oil came from a tree in Ecuador. The Ocotea oil has a light, cinnamon-like aroma and flavor. For centuries, this essential oil has been used for its anti-fungal properties and aromatic flavor. Studies show that Ocotea oil could control blood glucose levels and control food cravings.

Mint Essential Oil

This one is a very popular essential oil and commonly used to treat digestive problems. Unlike over-the-counter medications, you don't need to worry about the side effects of taking this oil frequently.

Overall, using essential oils is a great way to lose weight naturally, without experiencing any side effects. They're great for aromatherapy, massage, baths, and even ingesting them. These essential oils would help you achieve your weight loss goals while enjoying the other unique properties they have.

Nonetheless, they're ideal as scents in baths, massages, or aromatherapy because they could stimulate the brain and seep into the skin when used in baths. Likewise, by using a diffuser, you'd be able to use the essential oil around the house.

Caution: *When buying essential oils, make sure that you only opt for the genuine Therapeutic Grade ones, and not the diluted essential oils available in the market. Look for organic essential oils and use them with organic, pure carrier oils if you want to experience its optimum benefits.*

Essential Oils for Aromatherapy, Massage & Emotional Wellbeing

The efficient performance of the body and enhanced relaxation has been characterized by several factors. The most safe and recommended way to boost the overall well being of the body is through therapy, which tends to be more natural. Essential oils have been used for the remediation of any health and emotional problems in a person. It is used to aid in aromatherapy, massage and emotional wellbeing.

Essential Oils for Aromatherapy

You may be able to treat a number of physical problems through aromatherapy and relatively, every essential oil contains antiseptic properties that help in fighting any infections in the body. In addition, they help in killing fungi, bacteria, viruses, yeast or parasites.

Through Skin Absorption: The majority of the chemical ingredients of the essential oils contain molecules that weigh less than 1000m. It has been studied that any substance that has a molecular weight of less than 1000m can be absorbed through the skin. There are some essential oils that can be used in an aromatherapy mix for the sake of being absorbed into the tissues beneath.

Through Inhaling: It has been proved that the essential oils can be absorbed into the streams of the blood if they are inhaled. The senses of smell link with the limbic system of the brain, which is responsible for processing associations, memories and emotions.

Using essential oils for aromatherapy can impact the emotions. For instance, if you inhale Clary Sage, you may relieve the panic in you. On the other hand, the orange peel fragrance may boost the optimistic level of a person.

Essential Oils for Emotional Wellbeing

Essential oils can also help your emotional wellbeing.

Relaxation and Stress Relief: It has been studied that a small portion of lavender or Clary sage can assist in relieving yourself off from a stressful day. The Clary Sage is a great choice for boosting you up if you are emotionally upset or if you feel nervous. On the other hand, Lavender boosts the sleep and solves the insomnia cases.

Mental Enhancement: You might want a mental boost if you lack concentration or you are just tired. Peppermint, Rosemary, or Eucalyptus are great choices for mental stimulation. These oils will help to refresh your mind as well as inspiring you. With the Rosemary, it can assist to boost your concentration and attention level.

Essential Oils for Massage

The oils can be used also for massaging your body in order to boost your blood circulation and relax your mind as well.

Body Massage: For the overall body massage, you can use Lotion or Carrier oil, which will help in soothing your mind and entire body. If you want to use it for massaging your body, you will use a maximum of 6 drops or 2 to 3 teaspoons of the lotion or carrier oil like sunflower oil.

Facial Massage: The skin of your face is extra delicate and for that, it needs special care. The facial skin is also prone to display signs of toxic overload or stress. It is also more exposed to sun, wind and other pollutants in the atmosphere.

If you need to carry out a facial massage, it is best that you choose a suitable carrier oil. You will also need to use a lower amount of essential oil as compared to the amount you use for your body massage. Since the face is smaller, it is advised to use about 5ml of the overall solution mix for massaging it.

Localized Massage: The essential oils can also be applied in some areas, for instance around cramps (period pains or stomach), sprains or stiff joints. Such areas of pain need instant action, for that, the dilution ratio is usually lower than the one used in facial or body massage. All in all, you must ensure that you are using the right and recommended dosage.

Examples of Essential Oils to Use for Massage and Emotional Wellbeing

Some of the common and most used oils for massaging and emotional wellbeing include the following:

Lavender: It is an anti-depressant, anti-bacterial and anti-inflammatory oil that is used for various purposes. For instance, if you mix a few drops of lavender to sunflower oil and smear on your body, it can repel mosquitoes.

They can also chase away moths if they are dry and placed in the drawer or closet. They can mitigate stuffy nose if you add some drops to a humidifier. As you sleep, you may add some few drops on your pillow to boost your sleep.

Frankincense: This is a holy oil as it was presented to Jesus Christ by the wise men. It is used in several religious ceremonies for the sake of spiritual shield. The oil can also be added to soap or lotion to prevent pimples. It can also be used to cure and relieve burns, cuts, scrapes and rashes.

It is also believed to assist in offering a protective blockade in your aura, which avoids the intimidation of people's negativity. It may also be used to boost the immune system of children and enhance their sleep if they are mixed with coconut oil and rubbed on the kids' feet. You can rub some drops of Frankincense behind your ears, and around the wrist to alleviate stress. Using some drops on your handkerchief can also reduce the congestion in the nose if you inhale it, as it is well known to help in relieving asthma.

Peppermint: Over the years, peppermint has always been used to solve bad breath, relieve colic, ease tummy problems, headache, gas, indigestion and heartburn. Peppermint can also be used emotionally to allay anger, relieve depression and do away with fatigue. You can add some drops of Peppermint to your tea or coffee to lessen indigestion. Some drops applied at the back of the neck and around the shoulders can boost your energy throughout the day.

There are also other essential oils available, which can help in boosting your overall health, both physical and emotional. You may find the plant itself grown in the fields and pluck them, or you could buy a solution of the plants converted into oils. They will all perform the same functions, however, for the sake of faster absorption into the body system, you would best go for the oils. If you have the plant, you can add some water and boil them, then leave it to cool. The water should be in small amount in order to sustain the concentration required.

Essential Oils for Your Pet

It has been proven that essential oils can have very positive effects on pets for instance reducing anxiety, fighting infections, reducing inflammation and so much more. This is because the oils have numerous biological and powerful compounds that are useful to pets. These compounds usually have an impact on the pet's body system. The oils get into the pet's body through inhalation and by coming into contact with the skin.

Safe Essential Oils to use on Pets

Most of these are quite safe to use when giving a first aid to your pet or just for a short duration.

- Cardamom – This helps to get the pet's appetite back to normal and cures coughs, heartburn, and nausea. It is actually anti-bacterial.
- Lavender – Some small amount of lavender is quite useful when travelling with pets as it helps to calm them and make them sleep. Besides, it treats allergies, burns, and ulcers.
- Fennel - This is used to balance thyroid, pineal and pituitary glands in pets and to get rid of toxins. It is also quite helpful to the adrenal cortex.
- Helichrysum – It is a quick remedy to reduce bleeding when your pet has had an accident. This anti-bacterial oil helps to repair nerves and is essential if your pet is suffering from cardiac disease.
- Spearmint – This is a great remedy for weight reduction and balancing of metabolism. It is ideal for use when your pet is suffering from colic, diarrhea and nausea. It also stimulates the gall bladder and treats gastrointestinal problems in cats.

- Frankincense - This has been proven to be quite effective in cases of cancer in pets. This is because it is useful in the immune system and can reduce tumors or external ulcers.

Important Tips to Consider when Buying Essential Oils for Pets

It is necessary to use essential oils on your pets but there are few things to consider before you buy or even start using them. First and foremost never compromise on quality because the health of your pet matters most.

You have to research and ask a veterinarian before you get any oil for your pet. Always go for 100% pure natural Therapeutic Grade products. Always buy the right oils as advised by the veterinarian. In addition to that use the oils correctly. You should not use them in excess expecting to get quick results. Lastly and most important thing is to watch for any side effects as soon as you administer the oils to your pet.

How to Use Essential Oils on Pets

Pets are quite sensitive just as human beings. Therefore, once you buy the essential oil to use on your pet you should use them with caution. As much the oils offer a great remedy some of them can be quite dangerous because they contain adulterants or contaminates. Always use oils from reputable companies.

It is advisable to use diluted oils on pets because they are sensitive to smell and very strong smell can affect them. Never insist on using a given oil on your pet if you find them reacting negatively to the smell. It is also very important to use the right oil that is fit for a given species of your pet. In fact at times a given oil could work effectively on a cat but not a dog.

Some of these essential oils can cause serious problems on the liver and kidney to problems to the pets when used wrongly. This is because they are quite strong. Whenever using the essential oils ensure that they do not go into the eyes or directly into the skin unless it has to be applied to that area as directed.

It is advisable to keep these essential oils out of reach of children to prevent them from accidentally taking such. Always remember to wash your hands after touching these oils because they can be quite dangerous to adults too. It is recommended that you do not use a given oil for more than two weeks. This greatly reduces chances of the pet's organ reacting sensitively to a certain oil. You will actually have to take a break then continue administering the oil to your pet when necessary. However, in some occasions like cancer treatment you can use the oils longer as advised by a veterinarian.

Essential Oils for Personal Hygiene and Household Cleaning

Among other gifts of nature, essential oils particularly come with numerous health properties and benefits. This makes them ideal for all round use and their benefits encompass so diverse mediums like air and water. They are especially ideal for use on the body as their health benefits cover vital organs like the skin and brain. They also come with medicinal properties, which help heal scars and get rid of skin conditions like lesions and inflammation. They further go beyond this to even sooth emotions and the spirit, making them especially popular with physicians.

Essential oils are also ideal for use in general household cleaning as they come with many other properties that influence the surrounding environment.

Here is a detailed insight into the uses of essential oils:

Essential Oils for Personal Hygiene

Essential oils come with diverse benefits to the body. To users' advantage, these oils can be administered on the body in different ways. On the skin, these oils can be administered through bathing or direct application using soaked clothes and sponges. They can also be dispensed in the air to benefit the mind and spirit and soothe the body's breathing system.

Adding essential oils to bathing water

Essential oils are especially ideal for use with bathing water as this helps administer them evenly and wholly throughout the body.

However, caution is advised when using essential oils in bathing water as they are not entirely compatible with the water on their own. Seeing as it is these oils are not soluble in water, it is important that they first be mixed with salts or other emulsifier oils. This will help them get dissolved in the water and get dispensed on the skin better. It is also important to note that the high level of concentration of these oils requires that only a few drops be added to the bathing water. The water should also not be too hot as this may denature some of these oils, making them useless or even harmful.

Adding essential oils directly to the water will see them float, getting applied directly on the skin when bathing. This may not only affect their effectiveness, it may also affect your body negatively depending on their nature in hot water.

Applying essential oils directly on the skin

Essential oils can also be alternatively applied on the skin directly. Direct application is especially useful in situations where the skin has lesions, bruises or is suffering from skin conditions like inflammation. This is because essential oils come with diverse health benefits, and they are better harnessed and utilized through direct application in such needy cases.

Just as is the case with adding to bathing water, there are certain prerequisites that should be met before applying these oils on the skin. They are usually very concentrated, and as such should be dissolved using other emulsifier oils like Aloe Vera and hot water. They are applied on a soaked cloth and applied on the needy areas that basically comprise: aching muscles, bruises, inflammations and wounds among others.

Essential oils ideal for use on the skin

There are a lot of essential oils that come with diverse properties beneficial to the skin. They include:

- **Frankincense oil** - This oil comes with anti-inflammatory properties that make it ideal for treating skin conditions like acne and inflammation. It also comes with antibacterial properties, and has been shown to naturally induce even toning of the skin.

- **Lavender oil** - This oil is especially ideal for fighting off signs and effects of aging on the skin. Its properties are also beneficial in expediting the healing process of scars and wounds.
- **Carrot seed oil** - This oil has been shown to induce natural cell regeneration. This makes it ideal for administering on bruises, wounds and paining areas and muscles around the body. It also softens the skin, enhancing appearance and boosting confidence.

Administering essential oils through inhalation

The flexibility in essential oils also makes them ideal for use through inhalation. They are added to candle, electric or cool air diffusers, compressed with heat or simply added to hot water to dispense the fragrance into the air. Owing to their concentration, only about 10 drops of the essential oil is required for a standard sized room. Too much concentration of the fragrance in a room may cause nausea, headaches or dizziness.

However, when used in the right amounts, these oils can help in treating respiration conditions like colds, sinus infection, sore throat and coughs among others. Some of the best essential oils for inhalation include: eucalyptus, lavender, pine, frankincense, and thyme and tea tree.

Using Essential Oils for Household Cleaning

These oils are also beneficial in household cleaning as their medicinal properties make them excellent for fighting off bacteria and germs around the house. They also add a natural healing and soothing fragrance to the house, making it comfortable for living.

For use in household cleaning, these oils are added to cleaning water or mixed with other cleaning soaps and detergents. Their high concentration requires that only a few drops be added. After cleaning, the fragrance tends to linger in the house and on items that have had contact with the oils.

Some of the ideal essential oils to use for household cleaning include:

Lemon oil

Lemon oil comes with several conveniences when it comes to cleaning. For starters, it has antiseptic properties that make it ideal for removing stain and dirt off surfaces, clothes and other objects. Lemon oil also produces a sweet fragrance that keeps the house smelling cool and fresh.

Tea tree oil

Tea tree oil comes with tremendous cleanliness properties. For starters, it has been shown to have anti-bacterial and anti-fungal properties. This makes it ideal for cleaning rooms since it also leaves them safe as it eradicates germs.
It also leaves a nice medicinal smell that is soothing to the mind and which goes a long way in making the house even better habitable than before.

Peppermint oil

Peppermint essential oil is more ideal for adding fragrance to a room. The cool fragrance of the oil gives the house a fresh and cool smell. It however also comes with antiseptic properties that make it helpful when cleaning.

To the convenience of most people with different needs and preferences, essential oils have immense medicinal benefits and can be administered in the body in diverse ways. For safety when using these oils, ensure that all the guidelines are followed as different essential oils come with different properties.

Simple Essential Oil Recipes

Essential oils are one of nature's best-kept secrets. Besides smelling great, they can be used individually, or as blends for nearly everything under the sun, from repelling insects, to cleaning the toilet, to fighting infections. If you've been wondering how to blend these oils for your do-it-yourself projects, then these simple recipes will show you how.

Natural Toilet Scrub

You probably have found yourself buying different commercial toilet cleaners after watching them being advertised on your television. Yes, some of these products will leave your toilet sparkling clean, but they also contain toxic chemicals that put your family's health at risk if used in the long term. That is why it is better to formulate your own cleaner, using natural ingredients that are safe for your family. Here's how to make a natural toilet cleaner with essential oils.

Ingredients

A cup of distilled white vinegar

1 cup of baking soda

15 drops of tea tree oil

Directions

1. Mix the vinegar and the tea tree oil in a spray bottle and shake well.
2. Spray the mixture in your toilet bowl, as well as on the lid, seat and handle.

3. Wait for the mixture to settle for at least 30 minutes, sprinkle the baking soda inside the bowl, scrub with a toilet brush, and flush.
4. Using a clean and dry towel, wipe the vinegar solution from the seat, lid and handle.

This deodorizing formula uses tea tree oil's antibacterial properties to kill germs in the toilet.

Alternatively, you can also use the below recipe if you have stubborn stains that refuse to away even after using regular toilet cleaners.

Ingredients

1 cup of borax

1 cup of white vinegar

5 drops of lemon essential oil

10 drops of lavender essential oil

Directions

1. Mix all the ingredients in a bottle.
2. Flush the toilet to wet it.
3. Pour the mixture into your toilet bowl, and let it sit for several hours. If you can, allow it to sit overnight, ensuring that none of your family members use the toilet during the time.
4. Scrub the bowl thoroughly, and then flush the toilet to rinse.

It's worth noting that borax is not similar to boric acid, which is toxic. On the contrary, it is sodium tetraborate, which is a multi-purpose cleaner that deodorizes, whitens and removes stains. Just like baking soda, or table salt, borax can only be poisonous when used in very large amounts.

Borax and white vinegar are natural cleaning agents that help to disinfect and remove stains. On the other hand, lavender and lemon oils have anti-microbial and deodorizing properties, which help to kill germs and eliminating stale odors. Together, they'll leave your toilet extremely clean, and smelling nice too.

Natural Insect Repellant

If you love working in the yard, relaxing on the patio, or going for picnics, chances are, a mosquito, or other insects have bitten you. Did you know that you can make your own sprays using essential oils to repel these stubborn insects? The good news is that it only takes a few minutes to prepare the natural spray. Here's how:

Ingredients

2 tablespoons of vodka

2 tablespoons of either olive, jojoba, grapeseed, or almond oil (they contain natural insecticidal properties)

15 drops of rosemary oil

15 drops of lavender oil

15 drops of cedarwood oil

55 drops of lemon eucalyptus oil

Directions

1. Add the carrier liquids in a spray bottle, large enough to provide room for shaking.
2. Add the essential oils to the mixture, shake well and use.
3. For maximum effectiveness, reapply every few hours.

This homemade insect repellant works well on mosquitoes, flies, bugs and other annoying insects, so feel confident to tweak it to your liking. When not in use, store in a dark, cool place.

Homemade Dishwashing Liquid

Essential oils can also be used to make natural, chemical-free dish washing liquids that will get your dishes and sinks sparkling without digging too deep into your pocket. Here's a simple recipe to try:

Ingredients

1 tablespoon of borax

1 cup of water

1 tablespoon of grated bar soap (choose any natural bar soap you prefer)

10 drops of citrus essential oil

6 drops of eucalyptus oil

Directions

1. Heat the water until it boils.
2. Combine the grated bar soap and borax in a medium-sized bowl.
3. Pour the hot water over it, and whisk till the grated soap melts completely.
4. Let the mixture cool for about 6 hours, stirring occasionally.
5. Pour the formed gel in a bottle, add the essential oils, and shake well.
6. Your natural liquid soap is ready for use.

Citrus oil helps to remove grease, while the eucalyptus oil adds a fresh-smelling scent to the liquid, to make your dishwashing effective and enjoyable.

Natural Toothpaste

Why continue spending money to buy toothpastes when you can make your own at home using all natural ingredients? And the best part, it takes less than five minutes to prepare. Here's how:

Ingredients

10 drops of peppermint essential oil (use your favorite flavor)

1 tablespoon of fine sea salt (the minerals in the sea salt are great for your teeth, but you can leave it out if you find the taste too salty for you)

2/3 cup of baking soda

Filtered water

Directions

1. Mix together the baking soda, peppermint oil and sea salt.
2. Add a small amount of water at a time, and stir after each addition, till the paste reaches your desired co
3. That's it. No more excuses for having bad breath or stained teeth.

The above ingredients can make an equivalent of a 5.3 oz. tube full of toothpaste, so it will take a while before you make another one. To use, just wet your toothbrush, spread the toothpaste on the brush, and begin brushing. When not in use, store the preparation in a cool, dry place, preferably next to your toothbrush.

Natural Sinus Infection Treatment

If you've had a sinus infection before, then you know how awful it feels. The constant headaches, the stuffy nose, and loss of smell are symptoms that no one loves to go through. Fortunately, there are natural remedies that can help cure the infection for good. Essential oils, such as eucalyptus or peppermint oil, have anti-microbial properties, which makes them a powerful tool for treating sinus infections.

Ingredients

1 drop of peppermint or eucalyptus oil

1 tablespoon of coconut oil

Directions

Dilute the peppermint or eucalyptus oil in the carrier oil (coconut), and apply to the bridge of your nose. These essential oils are natural humidifiers, which help to open up nasal passages. Alternatively, you can also use frankincense to clear up the stuffiness.

Take advantage of the above simple, essential oil recipes, to make effective homemade products that are cheap and safe to use.

Conclusion

When used properly, essential oils can greatly improve your life by improving your overall health. These oils can often replace your medicine cabinet and your cleaning products if you would like them to. Doing this protects you from some of the harmful side effects of these products.

When choosing what essential oils to buy, quality of the most important factor. Price does not always mean the quality is there. Be sure to always choose Therapeutic Grade essential oils from trusted sources that have been in business for a while. Often, which brand to choose comes down to personal preference after you have found several that satisfied the quality standards.

If you do not know which brand to use, ask around for recommendations from friends and family. Personally I have used both Doterra and Young Living Essential Oils with amazing results, and I know others who have had great results with other brands of high quality essential oils.

Learning how to use your essential oils is a big step in taking charge of your health and emotional well-being. Congratulations on starting your journey!

Book 2

Essential Oils Recipe Guide For Health, Wellness & Household Use

By Grace Masters

Introduction

I want to thank you and congratulate you for downloading the book, "Essential Oils Recipe Guide for Health, Wellness and Household Use."

This book contains great recipes and solutions for using Essential oils in your everyday life.

Most people have a misconception about what exactly essential oils are with most people simply thinking that essential oils are only important for their smell. Did you know that there is more to essential oils than their sweet fragrance? Are you aware that you can use essential oils to relax, get rid of stress, help get rid of headaches, arthritis, and back pain among many other conditions? This book is the perfect guide for use of essential oils, as you will learn the different blends of essential oils you can make and how to use them for better health.

Thanks again for downloading this book, I hope you enjoy it!

Essential Oils: An Aromatic History

Essential oils are regarded as one of nature's best-kept secrets. Did you know that there are hundreds of different types of oils and blends being used every day for a range of applications? This means you can use essential oils for almost everything. Before we can move to using essential oils, it is prudent to know what exactly essential oils are. So what exactly are these 'essential oils?'

Essential oils can be described as concentrated, fragrant liquids that are extracted from the flowers, seeds, stems, roots, or bark of plants. Their extreme fragrances not only give plants their unique smells, but also ensure that the plant is protected from diseases and potential predators.

You might be thinking that the use of essential oils is a recent or modern phenomenon. However, that is not the case.

Egyptians

Throughout recorded history, essential oils have been used for numerous wellness, health and household applications. Egyptians were pioneers in the field of aromatic therapy, using essential oils to treat the sick. They also used them in religious festivities, in preparing their food, and even making themselves beautiful. They studied the properties of these compounds; learning their refinement and distillation processes.

Think about this, some of the most valuable goods transported along ancient trade routes were sandalwood, frankincense, cinnamon, and myrrh. I'm sure you have heard of frankincense and myrrh; these products are repeatedly referred to in many ancient religious texts. Frankincense, myrrh, and sandalwood were used in Egyptian embalming and cleansing rituals. These aromatic items were sometimes traded in for gold! That's right, gold. That shows you just how valuable these products were regarded.

Greeks

The Greeks quickly followed in the footsteps of the Egyptians, and began using essential oils for aromatherapy and therapeutic massages. Now, for those not familiar with aromatherapy, let me explain. Aromatherapy is a type of alternative medicine that uses natural plant oils/substances in order to enhance a person's mood, mental, or physical wellbeing. The aromas of the oils, once breathed in, are believed to stimulate brain function, and provide pain relief. Imagine inhaling the aroma of an essential oil, instead of popping painkilling tablets. Isn't the natural solution the best way to maintain vibrant health?

Romans

The Romans were also fond of using essential oils to enhance their personal health and hygiene. Not to be left behind, the Persians began to extract and distil essential oils from plants.

The Dark Ages

Essential oils were discovered to have anti-bacterial properties during the Dark Ages, and it is believed that French grave robbers used to apply it on their skin before they opened up the coffins of victims of the Bubonic Plague! The robbers practically immunized themselves against a disease that was virtually decimating the population! Clove and lemon oil were routinely used as disinfectants way before modern science evolved to become what it is today.

The Modern Age

Modern society has also picked up on the healing aspects of essential oils. This began in the early twentieth century, when the lab of a French chemist exploded, resulting in his hand getting severe burns. He immediately dipped it into what he thought was water. However, it was pure Lavender oil. He was so amazed at the pain-relieving effects it had on his wound that he continued applying it on his hand. In no time, the wound healed with minimal scarring. His subsequent studies on the healing properties of other essential oils laid the foundation of clinical use of essential oils. By the time the Second World War came around, soldiers were being treated using therapeutic-grade essential oils.

It is now clear that the use of essential oils is not something new. These natural compounds have been in existence for thousands of years. Modern medicine may have led to a reduction in their use, but they are still some of the most holistic and effective therapies around. There are numerous essential oil recipes that are available, and I intend to use this book to guide you in your quest to better understand essential oils. The recipes that are explored within this book will help you to make your own essential oils and enjoy the numerous benefits of these natural, aromatic substances.

What Exactly Are Essential Oil Compounds?

Essential oils are referred to as 'essential' because they contain the 'essence' of the aroma of the plant they originate from. Have you ever squeezed the peel of a mango or orange? What do you notice afterwards?

The aroma of the fruit still lingers on your fingers. Essential oils are volatile compounds that are instantly absorbed by the skin. That sweet fragrant residue that lingers on your hand is full of essential oils.

Properties and Applications

There are many and diverse uses of essential oils. As humans, our lives here on earth are dependent on plants, and they are responsible for our food, oxygen, clothing and overall health. What do you see when you look at a plant? Do you just focus on what is on the outside, or do you appreciate the complex nature that is hidden within? It's not all about the tasty fruits, you know.

The leaves, stem, flowers, bark, and roots all contain essential oils that can make a difference in your life. They contain the potent, natural, and healthy solution to a lot of the diseases and problems we experience in modern life. For example, did you know that just one drop of peppermint oil is equal to 25 cups of peppermint tea? Honestly, think of the potency of that single drop! Amazing, isn't it?

Many of these essential oils have antifungal, antidepressant, antibacterial, antiseptic, anti-inflammatory, and antiviral properties. They also have a great sensory impact on us, within minutes of applying or inhaling them. Their pleasurable aromas restore the body's natural state, enhancing your mood, emotional, and spiritual wellbeing.

Essential oils can be viewed as the plant's immune system, and in some instances, are just by-products of cellular metabolism. The reason they bear healing properties is because they have immeasurable organic compounds, for example vitamins, hormones, and other natural components. Essential oils may be stimulants or sedatives, meaning these organic components work on many different levels.

Ways of Administering Essential Oils

By now we all know how essential oils are beneficial to our physical and emotional wellness. It is your personal experience that will determine whether you use single oil or a blend of oils. Here are three ways of administering essential oils:

Aromatic Diffusion

It is a well-known fact that our sense of smell has a great influence on hormone stimulation and other physiological processes. It is your sense of smell that forms the basis of aromatherapy; the body has a predictable reaction to specific olfactory stimulants.

Some essential oils can be released into the air in order to provide a stimulating effect. On the other hand, others are more suited for calming and soothing you whenever you feel stressed or worked up. Think about it, you come home all tired and sore from the day's exertions, and you are greeted with a soothing scent of Bergamot-Geranium oil blend. You gradually start to feel the stress leave your body and energy flows through you once again. This is not magic or voodoo, this is nature's gift to you and it works wonders.

Apart from providing you with emotional wellbeing, essential oils can be used to purify the air around your home, eliminating both foul odors and certain harmful microbes. They can also come in handy when cleaning surfaces and doing laundry.

Topical Application

I mentioned before that the skin tends to absorb essential oils easily. The reason for this is the molecular structure of the oils, which allows you to apply them on your skin safely and experience instant benefits to those areas.

If you are into massages and beauty therapy, then essential oils can enable you to benefit from their calming and restorative properties. They also act as natural disinfectants, protecting the immune system and killing germs. By simply spraying it on your feet, arms or face, you benefit from full body protection from pathogens; remember how easy these compounds are absorbed into the bloodstream via the skin? That's how they work. When applying essential oils, remember to use carrier oils to dilute the oils as well as use skin patch test to know if you are allergic to a particular blend before you can proceed to applying on your whole body. Some common carrier oils include coconut oil, jojoba oil, grape seed oil, olive oil, and safflower oil.

Dietary Supplements

Using essential oils as dietary supplements can provide you with many health benefits. Some essential oils promote healthy development of cells, while others offer potent antioxidant benefits.

At this stage, I must warn you that not all essential oils you come across are meant for internal use. There are those that can be safely used for dietary applications, while there are those that should not. It is crucial that you check the labels for the appropriate dietary information. Those that can be used as dietary supplements MUST be labeled as such, and if so, make sure that you read the instructions carefully.

Grades of Essential Oils

So, while you may know how to use essential oils, do you know the kind of grade you need to use? There are many types of essential oils being marketed out there as 100% natural, organic and safe. I feel that you must be able to distinguish between the pure and beneficial oils and those that will clearly not do you any good. The industry itself does not have specific standards or regulations, so care is required on your part. Here are some distinctions in grades of essential oils:

1. Grade A (Therapeutic oils) – These are essential oils that are made from plants grown organically, and are distilled at a specific temperature through steam distillation.

2. Grade B (Food grade) – These essential oils may contain pesticides, fertilizers, or other synthetic additives. I would not recommend using this type of oils, as they are not pure.

3. Grade C (Perfume grade) – These essential oils have been known to contain impurities similar to those in Grade B oils. What the manufacturers do is use solvents

to obtain a greater yield of oil per harvest. These are commonly used in perfumes. I personally wouldn't recommend that you use this grade of oils because solvents are usually toI remember a time when the words 'natural' and 'organic' used to mean something. Nowadays, companies just misuse the terms to fool customers into buying their products.

4. Floral Water – This is actually a by-product of the distillation process of essential oils. Here's the catch: If it's obtained from distillation of Grade A essential oils, then it is of good quality. However, if it is obtained from low-grade oils or an improper distillation process, then the water is of poor quality. This grade of essential oil is commonly found in skin and hair products.

As a beginner, you probably aren't yet aware of what pure essential oils are supposed to smell like, right? Well, pure essential oils of therapeutic grade should have a balanced and broad aromatic profile, and should smell fresh. If what you experience is an overbearing and pungent scent, then you are most likely dealing with essential oils that have artificial chemical substitutes. The feel of a pure essential oil is also a sign. Pure essential oils should never be oily or slippery. They should be absorbed cleanly and totally by the skin.

It is important for you to keep a look out for the fake stuff that contains harmful chemicals. I remember when I started out using essential oils; it was difficult to tell what was pure and what wasn't. That's why you have to consult experienced users who can guide you on your path to achieving holistic health.

The Extraction Process

As an essential oils enthusiast, I think it is important that you have some understanding of how these aromatic and potent compounds are produced. As we have seen in the section above, how the essential oil is extracted determines its grade.

The low heat steam distillation technique is the most common technique used for extracting therapeutic-grade essential oils. Under this process, the pressurized steam is cycled through the plant matter resulting to essential oils being released into the vapor. Once the steam cools, the water and the natural oils will separate, thus enabling the oil to be collected in a pure form.

This process requires close monitoring of the temperature and pressure, as this is the only way of ensuring that the oils extracted are of the best chemical composition and of highest quality. If the heat and pressure used are too great, the potency and composition of the extract will be altered. On the other hand, if the heat and pressure applied are too low, the precious oil will not be released.

Other key factors that have to be considered are the proper selection of the appropriate plant, and harvesting of the correct parts of the plant at the right time.

The successful extraction of the essential oils is not just a science, but also a complex art. The distillers and plant growers must use their expertise and work as a team in order to ensure a quality product.

Here is a fact for you to ponder...

As many as 12000 rose blossoms are required to create just 5 ml of essential Rose oil (therapeutic grade).

I should also inform you that though steam distillation is the extraction method most commonly used, there is also a compression process that is used to extract citrus oils. It involves squeezing the oil from the plant.

Using Essential Oils: Safety Tips

As much as you now know about essential oils and the great things they can do in your life as well as how you can use them to benefit you, I must tell you that the benefits can only be maximized if purity is involved. Different countries have different government regulations concerned with the purity and quality of essential oils.

It is important that you know the source of your essential oils and how it is created in order to ensure effectiveness and safety for you and your family. It is also crucial that you understand how to use these essential oils. I have listed below some of the guidelines you should follow when using essential oils and essential oil supplements:

- Always make sure that you use essential oils that are unadulterated and of therapeutic-grade. Ensure that all instructions and warnings on the label are adhered to.

- When using essential oils topically, and you develop some kind of irritation or redness of the skin, make sure to apply some vegetable oil (for example olive oil) to the area affected.

- Please avoid using essential oils in the ear canal, the eyes, or in wounds that are open. In case of unintentional contact with the eyes, use vegetable oil to wash it out, but DO NOT use water.

- If you begin suffering from any extreme stomach, skin, or breathing problems, you should immediately stop using an essential oil.

- Essential oils should NOT be consumed orally unless it is a dietary supplement. In such a case, there should be a label that details the specific dietary supplement, with clear instructions and warnings.

- Make sure that you apply only a very little amount of oil on the skin of children. This is to test the child's sensitivity. Avoid applying the oil on the hands of the child as they may rub their eyes or mouth, thus transferring the oil.

- Always consult your doctor before using essential oils, especially if you are pregnant, suffering from some ailments, or have any doubts relating to essential oils.

With all the information that you have obtained from this book, it is still important that you keep in mind that essential oils are extremely potent compounds. Make sure that you are careful when dealing with them. If it is your first time experiencing essential oils, then I would recommend that you consult someone who has more experience with them. This way, you will better enjoy the rewards of using essential oils.

I am sure you are now ready to start using essential oils, so let's learn how you can use the different essential oils and achieve maximum benefit.

Blending Your Own Essential Oils

Have you ever considered blending your own essential oils? I remember when I first began using essential oils I had not figured out how to make blends so I just bought single oils as well as blends. It took a lot of time before I became confident in blending essential oils.

When you blend oils, ensure that the combination of oils are synergetic i.e. work together well enough to perform a specific function. For example, Eucalyptus oil and Lemon oil work well together to combat a dry cough.

There are a few factors that you have to consider when choosing to blend essential oils. We'll go through the steps so that you don't get confused, and it will seem easy once you get the hang of it. You need to ask yourself "what are my goals for blending the oils together? For what purpose am I going to use the blend?"

Let's assume that you want a blend that will enhance your mood and revitalize you. Now if you are a mom or dad, this would be great for morning use or in the middle of the afternoon, when you feel tired and worn out. It can also be sprayed in the kids' rooms when they are studying, keeping them alert and awake.

You will also need to choose which oils to incorporate into your blend; some are for external use, others internal, some are pure while others have additives. At this stage, it is important to know what the oils are for, the type you require, and then do some research on the companies that stock them.

If you want to make effective essential oils blend, kindly follow this process.

STEP 1: *Get the essential oils that you require*

There are minty, strong types like Peppermint, Rosemary, Pine, Eucalyptus, and Tea tree. There are also sweet spicy ones like Sage, Basil, and Bergamot.

STEP 2: *Blending the essential oils*

Now that you have narrowed down your choices according to your needs and goals, we can start blending. The recommendation is to begin with 10 drops of essential oils in total, so that you don't waste precious oils. Please note that there is no dilution at this stage.

STEP 3: *"Rest" the essential oil blend*

This simply means that you allow the blend to sit for about 24 hours so that the compounds can mix and merge.

STEP 4: *The test*

Now that the essential oil blend is ready, take a whiff and see what it smells like. You can also try diluting the blend using a carrier oil e.g. Jojoba or massage oil (if you are applying it on the skin). I would recommend that you pick carrier oils that do not have strong scents. The ratio of dilution is up to you if the blend is for aromatherapy. Otherwise, the exact recipes for various health problems are outlined in the chapters below.

Make more of your favourite blend and bottle it for future use. If a particular scent doesn't appeal to you, just start all over and combine different oils of your choice, or vary the amounts. It truly is a world of endless possibilities!

Remember the safety tips I outlined previously, as you are dealing with concentrated compounds that may be harmful if misused. The following chapters describe in detail essential oil recipes (single oils and blends) that are used for different applications.

Essential Oil Recipes For Health

The recipes below include use of single oils and blends (combination of different essential oils). I have categorised them according to the disease or ailment they treat.

1. Recipe for Diarrhoea/Salmonella/ E-Coli

1 drop Cinnamon Bark oil

Water

Put one drop of cinnamon bark oil in a cup of plain water, and drink the mixture several times daily. Cinnamon bark is known to have antiviral properties.

2. Recipes for Headaches

25 drops Sweet Marjoram

25 drops Lavender

6 drops Peppermint oil

Massage oil

Place the essential oils in an empty bottle and add massage oil (the massage oil acts as a carrier oil). Rub the mixture on the temples, neck, and forehead.

3. Recipe for Bloating and Constipation

3 drops Red Mandarin oil

1 drop Peppermint oil

Mix the oils and rub on your stomach. The oils will be absorbed through the skin and into the bloodstream, triggering the release of gas.

4. Recipes for Dry Cough

Method 1

4 drops Eucalyptus oil

4 drops Lemon oil

2 tablespoons honey

Glass of warm water

Mix the oils with the honey. Place one teaspoon of the mixture in a glass of warm water and sip it slowly.

Method 2

4 drops of Thyme

4 drops of Eucalyptus oil

1 teaspoon of olive oil

Combine the Eucalyptus oil and the Thyme, and then dilute them in the olive oil. Massage this mixture on the chest and back.

5. Recipe for Lice Removal

1 tablespoon Jojoba oil

7 drops Rosemary oil

8 drops Geranium oil

Mix the oils then massage into the hair and scalp before you sleep. Use this mixture every night until all the lice are eliminated. You can even wrap a towel around the head for the duration of the night.

6. Recipe for Ear Infection

2 drops Lavender oil

3 drops Tea Tree oil

1 drop Thyme

1 teaspoon Massage oil

Add the ingredients together and apply the mixture around the ears, jaws and down the neck. This will drain the lymph nodes, eliminate the infection and ease the pain.

7. Recipe for Menstrual Cramps

5 drops Clary Sage oil

15 drops Thyme oil

10 drops Chamomile oil

4 tablespoons Massage oil

Pour the massage oil into a bottle, and add the essential oils. Shake the bottle, and then apply the mixture on the abdomen (begin near the navel) in circles. Perform the process 3 times.

8. Recipe for Constipation

5 drops Peppermint oil

10 drops Lemon oil

15 drops Rosemary oil

Combine the essential oils and then dilute the blend in 2 tablespoons of vegetable or massage oil. Working in an anti-clockwise motion, massage the mixture over the lower part of the stomach three times every day.

9. Recipe for Athlete's Foot

1 drop of Lavender oil

2 drops Tea tree oil

5 drops massage oil

Mix all the ingredients and apply the blend to your feet and toes. Do this at least two times a day.

10. Recipe for Allergies

2-4 drops of Lavender oil

2-4 drops of Lemon oil

2-4 drops of Peppermint oil

Local raw honey

Mix honey with oils and swallow or add to hot tea or hot water and drink. Repeat daily or as needed for allergy symptoms.

Note: *Use only food grade essential oils when ingesting.*

11. Recipe for Stuffy Nose

1 drop of Lavender oil

Put the oil on your finger and rub on just inside or below each nostril. Alternatively, you can swipe your oiled finger on the inside of your cheek.

Note: *Use only food grade essential oils when ingesting.*

Essential Oil Recipes For Wellness

These recipes help to resolve minor ailments, boost cognitive functions, and elevate your mood.

1. Recipe for Effective Studying

> 1 drop Peppermint oil
>
> 5 drops Rosemary
>
> 7 drops massage oil
>
> Mix the ingredients in your palms and rub onto your face, neck, and hands in order to release the fragrant properties that boost focus and alertness.

2. Recipes for Stress

Method 1:

> 10 drops Geranium oil
>
> 30 drops Bergamot
>
> 10 drops Ylang Ylang
>
> Mix the Essential oils in a bottle and add massage oil. Rub the mixture on your skin, near the nose to inhale the aroma. You will instantly feel a calming effect.

Method 2:

> 2 ounces of sesame seed oil
>
> 2 drops of Spikenard oil
>
> Mix the ingredients and massage onto the forehead, the rear of the neck, and the scalp. This will soothe you and relieve the stress.

3. Recipes for Congestion

1 drop Peppermint oil

Hot water

Place one drop of peppermint oil in a bowl full of hot water and inhale the steam.

4. Flu and Sinus Blend

6 teaspoons of Niaouli oil

3 teaspoons of Rosemary oil

3 teaspoons of Pine oil

2 teaspoons of Lavender oil

2 teaspoons of Lemon oil

4 ½ cups of alcohol (90%)

Combine all the above ingredients together. Put 3 teaspoons of the blend into a bowl of 6 cups of boiling water then inhale the steam.

Place 3 drops of the blend in bath water and dip into the water.

Add 1-2 drops of the blend into a footbath.

5. Digestive Support Blend

10 drops of Cardamom

10 drops of Ginger oil

5 drops of Tarragon oil

Blend the essential oils together while shaking vigorously. This blend can be placed in a diffuser and sprayed, massaged onto the abdomen in clockwise strokes or 3 drops of the blend added to a cup of tea.

6. Recipe to Lower High Blood Pressure

30 drops Clary sage

10 drops Sweet Marjoram

10 drops Lemon oil

10 drops Ylang Ylang

Combine the ingredients in a bottle and then fill it with massage oil. Apply the blend to the skin, where it will be absorbed to relieve the effects of high blood pressure.

Using Essential Oils For Weight Loss

Losing weight requires much more than just essential oils, but they can make a big difference when added to an exercise and a lifestyle change. Consider this for a moment...

Any form of health improvement requires a holistic approach that factors in digestive issues, stress, diet, exercise, habits, the body's immunity, and even your spiritual/emotional wellbeing.

Most people fail with their weight loss efforts because they fail to address all the underlying issues. Dealing with only one or a few of the contributory factors without resolving others results in failure. A holistic approach that incorporates essential oils can be of great benefit when you want to lose weight, as long as you connect with your mind, body, and spirit.

Here are some of the essential oils that can help in weight loss:

Grapefruit

Grapefruit has been proven to help combat overeating, toning, and cellulite. It also elevates your mood, which is an integral part of exercise and body image.

Lemon

Lemon gradually eliminates toxins in the body, while raising your levels of energy. It uplifts your spirits and emotions, which helps you to exercise for weight loss and also in self-acceptance.

Peppermint

Peppermint is effective in curing any digestive problems, excites the mind and deals with Candida (tends to be a factor in weight gain). It also elevates your mood, thus motivating you in your fitness goals.

Ginger

Ginger increases levels of energy, stimulates the system, and keeps the body warm. It tends to create a sense of spiritual and emotional strength that allows you to break through exercise plateaus and work harder to lose weight.

Cinnamon

It has been shown that cinnamon has a positive effect on all the other essential oils used in weight loss. It boosts blood circulation, cleanses the body, and boosts the immune system. It is also said to improve your outlook on life, and your own body image.

Essential Oils For Household Use

If you are keen on using essential oils for making homemade cleaning products but are unsure of where to begin, then read on.

The three main reasons for using essential oils for household use are:

- The strong scents that are produced by these strong, fragrant compounds.

- Some essential oils have unique chemical constituents that make them good cleaning products, e.g. citrus essential oil.

- Some essential oils have antiseptic or disinfectant properties, e.g. Tea Tree oil.

Please note that these recipes do not instruct you on the number of drops, but instead give you ratios to use. This is because it will depend on which homemade cleaning products you are using and which essential oil is more prominent.

1. Citrus fruit blend

This is for stain-removal and cleaning purposes.

3 parts Lemon oil

1 part Bergamot oil

1 part Lavender oil

2. Flowery and fresh blend

Equal proportions of Lemon and Lavender oils. This is for a sweet aroma.

3. Herbal blend

2 parts Eucalyptus oil

4 parts Rosemary oil

5 parts Lavender oil

4. Minty blend

Equal proportions of Eucalyptus and Peppermint oils.

This imparts a good scent in the cleaning products and cures colds and congestion.

5. Natural Sink and Bathtub Cleaner Recipe
This recipe is pretty simple and easy to make and is specifically meant for sinks and bathtubs. The ingredients used to make this recipe are skin friendly and quite effective in killing bacteria.

1 cup Baking Soda

20 to 30 drops of the Thieves Essential Oil Blend

In a small bowl (mixing bowl), place baking soda enough to clean all your bathtubs and sinks. Add a considerable amount of Thieves essential oils for cleaning, (about 25 drops); stir well until all the ingredients are uniformly mixed. Finally, pour the mixture into a 6 or 8oz glass jar and close it tightly.

Sprinkle the mixture lightly into sinks and/or bathtubs; give it a few seconds and then scrub thoroughly before rinsing with plenty of water.

6. Bathroom and Kitchen Purifying Spray

This recipe is for cleaning kitchen table cabinets and bathrooms mirrors, dressing tables and detergent cabinets.

1 quart spray bottle

3 drops of Rosemary

4 drops lemon

3 drops Eucalyptus

4 drops Lavender

Fresh water

Add substantial water into a spray bottle, add each and everyone item of the above listed essential oils for cleaning and shake thoroughly.

Spray the cleaner on all surfaces in bathroom and kitchen then wash normally. Additionally, this spray can also be used as an air freshener and is effective in keeping away bugs.

7. Window Cleaner

For window and mirror cleaning, you will need a somewhat strong cleaner with bleaching power. Window cleaner discussed here is quite easy to make and use.

1 Quart spray bottle

1 cup white Vinegar

12-16 drops of the Lemon Essential Oil

In a clean spray bottle, add vinegar, water and all the above-mentioned oils then shake thoroughly.

Spray the cleaner on the window and mirror then wipe using a soft rag.

8. Stain Remover Recipe

Use 2 to 3 drops of the lemon essential oil on the target stain, give it a couple of seconds and then rub off with a clean piece of cloth, alternatively, instead of rubbing it with a clean piece of cloth, throw it into your normal laundry cycle.

9. Tiny Ant Repellant

This essential oil household recipe is for keeping away annoying ants running after sugar in kitchen cabinets and some bugs mostly found in closets.

1 quart spray bottle

15-20 drops of your Purification Essential Oil

10 drops of Peppermint essential oil

Water

Fill the spray bottle with some water until its full, add the listed essential oils and stir thoroughly.

Simply Spray the Repellant in cabinets and closets. Alternatively, you can spray the repellent in the cotton ball and then set it right in the corner of the cabinet. The peppermint in this cleaner will also deter rodents such as rats.

10. Dishwasher and Dish Essential oil Detergent

Many dishes and dishwashers are made using stainless material. To extend their durability, it is mandatory that you take good care of them. This recipe, apart from cleaning, is also quite good in retaining your utensils and appliances quality.

Liquid castile soap

Water

Few drops of your essential oil (any of your choice but not lemon)

In your spray bottle, add 1 cup of fresh water. Add another cup of liquid castile soap, and few drops of any essential oil, before shaking.

Use this detergent the same way like other dish detergent and be sure to rinse thoroughly before drying the dish/dishwasher dry.

11. Floor Cleaner

Floor is quite simple to wash. All you need is a detergent capable of stripping out dirt and with some disinfectant powers. To start with, combine one part white vinegar with slightly warm water in a bucket and use a rag o a mop to scrub the floor. Once the floor dries up, spray some purifying spray from recipe number 6 above.

12. Essential oil Hand Soap

This is crucial since you will require it every time you are done with cleaning the bathroom or kitchen or even doing the laundry.

Mix water with liquid castile soap and a few drops of your essential oils for cleaning, preferably lavender or lemon. Pour it on your hands and massage your hands until there is enough foam. Rinse your hands with cold water before drying.

Conclusion

We have come a long way in our journey to educate ourselves about essential oils, and I hope you have picked up information that will not only benefit you now, but for a lifetime.

Book 3

Essential Oils Guide For Cleansing, Oil Pulling & Health

By Grace Masters

Introduction to Essential Oils

From magazine articles to beauty blog topics, it seems that essential oils are the phrase on the tip of everyone's tongues these days. By now, you're probably wondering what all the hype is about. Truthfully, there's good reason for all of the attention that essential oils are receiving lately: they are all-natural sources of wondrous wellness properties that can provide detoxification for your body, as well as other beneficial impacts.

To put it simply, essential oils are naturally-occurring substances found in plants, which embody the valuable characteristics of that plant, such as fragrance or medicinal purposes. In other words, the essential oil is the life force of the plant, captured in an applicable liquid form. Many essential oils have myriad advantages, including antifungal, antibacterial, and antiviral properties. They can be easily absorbed and promote nourishment within the body. Best of all, they're entirely natural and do not come with any of the harmful risks or side effects associated with many everyday medications and processed substances.

Does Your Body Need a Detox? The Benefits and Advantages of a Natural Cleanse

Every day, your body is exposed to an abundance of toxins. You may think that you're leading a healthy lifestyle, but even those of us who do our best to eat well, get adequate sleep, and avoid polluted environments are still prone to the exposure of free radicals and other toxins. You could even be ingesting harmful, unnatural ingredients in the processed foods that you eat.

For instance, there typically aren't any specific regulations that must be met for a food product to advertise itself as being "all-natural" on the label - chances are that even if you opt for these kinds of foods, you're still consuming processed components. Just because a food contains *some* natural ingredients doesn't necessarily mean that other components of the products aren't processed. Likewise, even produce puts you at risk; unless you're consistently consuming wholly organic fruit and vegetables, you're likely to be ingesting some trace levels of pesticides or other harmful additives.

Even the air we breathe presents harmful risks to our bodies. From pollution to harsh cleaning products, toxins are present everywhere we turn. As hard as we may try to live an all-natural life, we simply cannot control every aspect of our environment, and we truly live in an inorganic world. We can only control our immediate surroundings and the impact that *we* create on the environment - unfortunately, free radicals and other harmful toxins are a reality in today's society, no matter how much we strive to make our own carbon footprint as small as possible. Of course, these pollutants have a negative impact on our bodies, and it's probably worse than we even realize.

Luckily, essential oils have the power to rid your body of these toxins. Not only can they flush your systems in a healthful manner, but they can also promote an even hormonal balance, enhance liver functionality, support your adrenal system, and encourage urinary health. An essential oil cleanse can leave your body's systems, and especially your digestive tract, feeling refreshed and highly functional.

Still, you may feel as though everything in your body is functioning as it should. Perhaps you're eating as healthfully as you can, and you haven't really experienced any digestive issues. Yet, simply feeling healthy *enough* isn't an indication in itself that you don't need a detox. Signs that are seemingly insignificant - chronic halitosis (also known as bad breath) or even headaches, for example - can be indicators that your body may need a refresher. If you become ill frequently, develop skin irritations, allergies, and even experience regular fatigue, there's a strong chance that you may benefit from an essential oil cleanse.

Oftentimes, we neglect to realize that the source of inflammation, irritation, and other health maladies are a direct result of our environment, or the toxins we've been exposed to. By ridding ourselves of these toxins, we enable our bodies to function at their best. As a result, you'll feel more energized, and most likely, you'll be even healthier than you even thought possible.

Because essential oils are highly concentrated, they are extremely powerful. The efficacy is greater in essential oils than in alternative forms of nourishment. For example, tangerine oil will have a higher concentration of the vitamins and minerals than what's found in the fruit itself, because it's been intensified into a much stronger form.

When you use essential oils to enhance your body's functionality, you'll also be more likely to reduce some of the other factors that can bog you down, such as stress and anxiety. The mind and body are intertwined quite intensely, and alleviating any issues within your physical wellbeing will only enhance your mental and emotional health. Some individuals have even been able to alleviate or overcome depression, thanks in part to the use of essential oils in their everyday routine.

If you're experiencing any of the physical (or even psychological) issues listed above or simply want to restore your body to its maximum level of functionality, then you're the perfect candidate for an essential oil cleanse. When performed properly, there are virtually no health risks, and the potential rewards are entirely worthwhile.

How to Cleanse and Detoxify Your Body with Essential Oils

As we mentioned previously, essential oils are extremely potent. While this is beneficial in terms of their myriad healing aspects, it also means that essential oils should almost never be consumed directly (without being diluted) or applied in raw form to the skin. Oftentimes, oils must be combined with other substances, such as carrier oils, alcohols, waxes, or other means of dilution, before ingestion or application. Again, because essential oils are highly concentrated, your body may not be able to handle the potency and you could experience rashes or irritation if directly exposed to an essential oil that hasn't been diluted. That's why so many essential oil brands sell blends, instead of oil that's 100% concentrated.

There are a few means by which you can expose your body to an essential oil in a healthy and safe way and still reap all of the benefits associated with the oil. Many oils can be applied topically, but as we mentioned above, it's a good idea to dilute them if they haven't already been blended down (especially if you have sensitive skin). In fact, if your skin is prone to redness or rashes, you may want to dilute the consistency of your essential oil with a carrier even further, just to be safe. Diluting doesn't diminish the efficacy of an essential oil's benefits, so it never hurts to do so.

Later on, we'll discuss in greater detail the different types of oils you can use to target specific health concerns. For now, it's important to know that some essential oils are more effective when applied to the skin, but may need to be diluted heavily. If in doubt, your best bet is to dilute an oil before applying to the skin with a carrier oil such as coconut oil. You'll want to use a ratio of about three drops of coconut oil for every one drop of the essential oil.

There are different methods for applying an essential oil directly to your skin. For one, you can administer the oil directly over the area of concern. Applying an essential oil to the abdomen, lower back, or anywhere else that you feel a cleanse might be appropriate will help to target that area first.

Another (and perhaps more enjoyable) means of administering an oil is massaging it into the skin. Wherever you begin from, you should work your way in towards the heart from your extremities.

The most effective way of topically applying essential oils is to place them on the reflex points on the hands, feet, and ears. Applying essential oils to the feet is perhaps the best option - it allows for quicker absorption into the bloodstream, and that area of your body is less likely to develop any kind of irritation if your skin is sensitive to the oil.

You can also ingest essential oils, but again, we urge you to take caution and dilute the oil when in doubt. It's important to make sure that any essential oils you plan to use internally are of food grade level or higher quality. *Never* ingest any essential oils that are not at least food grade, and if the directions do not call for ingesting, don't guess; it's best to apply topically when in doubt. While some essential oils can be added directly to water - peppermint and lemon, for example - there are others that must be diluted with honey or dissolved in capsules. For these, you can add one drop of the essential oil to a teaspoon of honey, or follow the oil's directions regarding capsules. There are many different types of essential oils that can also be incorporated into food preparation, as well, such as oregano or rosemary.

Quick Cleanse for Beginners

If you're new to essential oils, we suggest trying out a short-term cleanse that will ease you into the holistic world of healing.

First, you'll want to decide which essential oil you'd like to use. While you could create a blend that targets multiple areas of the body and allows for a thorough cleanse, we advise starting slowly, especially if you've never used essential oils in the past.

Peppermint oil is typically a safe bet for beginners. It has detoxifying properties and is generally a bit gentler than other varieties. Laurel oil is another popular choice, thanks to its antioxidant rich properties; also, it stimulates digestion and acts as an expectorant. Juniper oil, grapefruit oil, and lemon oil are also great detoxifiers.

Once you've chosen your desired oil, you will need to select a brand of essential oil to purchase. Nowadays, essential oils are much easier to acquire than they once were, and can often be purchased online or in natural markets or specialty stores. Just make sure that regardless of the brand you choose, you read the directions thoroughly, including whether or not the oil must be diluted, and whether it's intended for ingestion or topical use only. Again, we recommend seeking out food grade essential oils specifically if you intend to ingest them.

Some popular brands of essential oils are Beeyoutiful, Mountain Rose Herbs, NOW, and Young Living. You can choose the oil brand that fits your needs and your budget best.

Once you've made your purchase, you may wish to perform a "test" prior to beginning the cleanse by applying a very small amount of the essential oil (again, dilute it if necessary) directly to your skin. Wait for a period of 24 hours, and discontinue use if you notice any itchiness, redness, or irritation.

After you've performed a preliminary test and made sure that your skin doesn't develop a bad reaction, you can begin the quick cleanse. Depending on your selected method of application and the directions provided by your essential oil, you can apply 3-5 drops of the oil to your feet, ingest the oil via a capsule, or drink it directly after dropping it into a glass of water. The oil may also be safe to ingest with honey, or you might be able to apply it with a carrier oil. Again, take caution to read the instructions provided and never ingest or apply an essential oil in a way other than the directions recommend.

Also, there's no harm in starting out at a slower pace to familiarize your body with the presence of an essential oil. You may even want to use a lower dosage than the recommended amount at first, so as to break yourself in. Your body may experience a lot of changes during the time when you first begin your cleanse - this is natural and to be expected. You're flushing out your systems, which is beneficial for your body, but it's best to do this gradually and slowly instead of going to extremes right away. If you are satisfied with the results and don't experience any signs of distress within your body, give yourself at least seven days before beginning a new phase or moving on to the long-term cleanse.

Beginners should embark on a seven-day cleanse for best results. During this phase, you should also aim to consume a generous amount of water throughout the day - you should probably drink a bit more than you normally would. Likewise, for best results, you should also try to balance your diet effectively, consuming only organic fruits and vegetables, if possible. While this type of dietary regimen doesn't fit perfectly into every individual's lifestyle, it may be the best option for providing optimal detoxification benefits. Remember, your goal here is to rid your body of toxins, so continuing the consumption of processed foods throughout this period could hinder your body's ability to cleanse itself. At the very least, try to avoid inorganic animal food products and processed or unrefined carbohydrates. If you can manage it, your best bet would be to avoid prepackaged food altogether.

Gentle Long-Term Cleanse

If you have experience with essential oils or have tried out our quick cleanse and want to move on to a long-term routine that will effectively detoxify your body over an increased timespan, then we recommend using the method below to reap substantial health benefits as possible. By extending the period of time in which you use the essential oils, you can maximize the beneficial effects they will have on your body and ensure a total cleanse that will gradually flush the toxins in a healthful, gentle manner.

First, you'll want to select the essential oil that you'll be using. You're going to either ingest (if it's safe and food grade level, per the oil's instructions) or topically apply this oil for the next 28 days, so make sure that it's something you'll be comfortable with for long-term use. Your best bet it to select an essential oil blend that is intended specifically for detoxifying purposes. Below, you'll find a list of popular essential oils used in detoxifying blends:

- Cilantro - This essential oil has a high level of antioxidants, and is an effective detoxifier, thanks to its ability to remove heavy metals and lead from the body.
- Geranium - It's extremely effective in regulating hormones and promoting kidney and liver function. Geranium is also a diuretic, which makes it an ideal contender for any cleanse.
- Rosemary - This antioxidant-rich essential oil is also antibacterial, can prevent fatigue, and supports the endocrine system.
- Tangerine - It's known for promoting digestive health, and helps to cleanse the colon and liver. In addition, it has anti-inflammatory properties.
- Juniper - Originating from juniper berries, this essential oil is a great source of antioxidants, can be used as a diuretic, and aids in digestion. It can also banish water weight and flush toxins from the body.

After selecting your blend, you will be ready to begin the long-term detox cleanse.

Every day, you'll either apply the essential oils topically (per the directions) or ingest them, as long as you've selected the type that can be consumed. You only need to use essential oils once per day, and it's best if you do it in the morning so as to wake your body's internal systems and get them to start working right away.

While your dietary requirements and overall lifestyle will most likely determine what you eat during this cleanse, know that your diet is going to have an effect on how well the cleanse works for you. Above all else, you're going to need to drink a significant amount of water throughout the time of your detox.

To see the best results, it's a good idea to avoid all processed foods throughout the time of your cleanse. Because you're ridding your body of toxins, you won't want to put any more in to your systems at this time - that could throw the entire detox off balance. If you can't go totally organic, sticking only to pesticide-free fruits and veggies for the full twenty-eight days, feel free to include pastured meat, including pork and chicken, and organic eggs in your diet. That way, you'll be sure to stay full enough so that you can last through the twenty-eight day period without ever becoming too hungry. You can also incorporate organic butter, olive oil, and coconut oil into your diet. These will provide healthy fats and help ward off hunger.

It's best to avoid wheat, sugar, grains, most dairy, and all processed foods during this time. An all-natural diet will work most efficiently to restore your body to its best level of functionality. Keep in mind, though, that you don't need to deprive yourself at all - yes, you're reaping the benefits of a cleanse by detoxifying your body, but that doesn't mean that you have to go hungry.

Again, be sure to continue to drink plenty of water during this time. Feel free to continue exercising if you normally do, but don't begin any new intense workout regimens during your cleanse period. After the 28 day period is complete, take at least seven days off from the cleanse before beginning another detox cycle. You can continue to eat healthfully, but it's recommended that you give your body's systems some time to let the benefits of the cleanse sink in.

Oil Pulling with Essential Oils

One method of using essential oils that doesn't require any application or ingestion is oil pulling. It's gained popularity in recent years, and for good reason: the countless benefits of this practice are overwhelming. So for anyone who's new to the practice or could use an explanation, oil pulling is the act of swishing essential oils around in your mouth to expose your body to the helpful benefits they offer.

Although oil pulling is reappearing in today's society, it has actually been in practice for thousands of years. The exercise began in ancient India and was used to cure common health maladies, and was regarded as a useful healing method by natural health practitioners during that time. Today's health practitioners and researchers are still completing research regarding the benefits of oil pulling, but we can only speculate that thousands of years of history during which the practice was relied on must hold some value.

Oil pulling is an inexpensive, painless way to enhance your wellness. For those who are hesitant to try an essential oil cleanse, we suggest starting here with oil pulling instead. It will expose your body to the benefits of essential oils in a gradual, gentle manner, and you can go at your own pace by controlling the amount and frequency within your oil pulling practice.

Benefits of Oil Pulling

Swishing essential oils around in your mouth may sound a bit strange to you - many of us are accustomed to using mouthwash, but have never experimented with other liquids. We bet you'll change your mind after reading this, though.

For one thing, swishing with essential oils can detoxify your body by removing the harmful bacteria and toxins that live in your mouth and lymph system. Specifically, the essential oils can target mouth-related health issues, including periodontitis and gingivitis.

Most importantly, however, is the fact that the health of your mouth is directly related to your overall wellbeing. Your gums are essentially an open gateway to your bloodstream - in other words, any toxins and bacteria that reside in your mouth have easy access to your bloodstream, and therefore, your entire body. Of course, you're not knowingly putting toxic chemicals or harmful substances in your mouth, but exposure to processed foods, germs, free radicals, and pollution in general can put you at risk.

Moreover, common mouth-related health issues, such as gingivitis and periodontitis, have the potential to wreak greater havoc on your body. Periodontitis, which typically begins with gingivitis, may be associated with heart disease and diabetes. Disease prevention is perhaps the greatest reason to take care of your mouth; especially since heart disease is often linked with potentially fatal issues such as stroke and heart attack.

Even if you consider your oral health habits to be excellent, oil pulling is an additional way to truly boost your regimen into high gear. While greater overall health is one incentive for practicing daily oil pulling, consider this: daily oil pullers have also experienced migraine relief, reduced allergies, and even mental health improvement. Oil pulling also has the potential to boost your metabolism, heal mouth sores, whiten teeth, and fasten loose teeth. In the next section, we'll discuss even more specific health concerns that can be addressed through the use of various essential oils.

If you're curious about how the oil pulling process works, it's actually quite simple. When you swish the oil around in your mouth, it begins to mix with saliva, thereby activating enzymes within your mouth. These enzymes then are able to draw toxins out of your gums, and from your bloodstream. The oil becomes thinner as you work it around in your mouth.

How to Practice Oil Pulling with Essential Oils

The practice of oil pulling is very simple, yet extremely effective. There are different types of essential oils which target specific health concerns, so you don't always have to use the same type of oil every day, especially if you'd like to address various issues.

Oil pulling is most effective when practiced first thing in the morning, prior to brushing your teeth. The benefits are maximized when you perform oil pulling on an empty stomach. You'll need to swish for about twenty minutes, so feel free to perform oil pulling while completing other activities. Many people choose to do their oil pulling while in the shower; just be careful not to swallow it.

You can select your essential oil for pulling from a variety of brands and types, as long as they are food grade level and recommended for internal use. Even though you won't be swallowing the essential oil, it's important to make sure that it's safe enough to be used in your mouth.

Beginners should use about one teaspoon of essential oil. Over time, you can increase the amount to about two teaspoons, and then eventually one tablespoon. You can also gradually increase the frequency of your oil pulls. At first, start out by pulling only in the morning, but as you continue use, feel free to increase the frequency and complete it up to three times daily if you're suffering from an acute health condition.

While simply swishing the oil around is effective, oil pulling is practiced best by using a specific method. The reason it's called pulling, in fact, is because you should sip and suck the oil, essentially "pulling" it through your teeth. This pulling method effectively extracts toxins and bacteria from your mucous membranes. As you swish, the oil will change in consistency and may even take on a milky hue.

Twenty minutes may seem like a long time for swishing, but the timeframe is perhaps the most crucial aspect of oil pulling. Research shows that this is the necessary amount of time for all of the toxins to be pulled from the mouth's cavities, yet it's not too long so that the waste will be redistributed back into the body.

Once you've swished for twenty minutes, spit the oil out into your trash can. Certain types of oils can cause a drainage block and are unsafe for septic systems. Make sure to spit all of it out completely, and avoid ingesting any of the oil residue; it's filled with toxins and bacteria.

After you've extracted the oil, it's important to clean your mouth thoroughly. Begin by rinsing your mouth with warm water, and brushing with a protective blend afterwards. There are a few different antibacterial blends available that will further ensure your oral health, from brands such as Ora Wellness and On Guard.

In some cases, you may be able to find essential oil blends that benefit various parts of the body and its systems. Many people target specific issues or concerns by using the appropriate essential oil to alleviate them. The list below reveals the many uses of some common essential oils.

Lemon - While it's an overall detoxifier, lemon oil contains a significant amount of antioxidants. It can also be used as an antiseptic and help to alleviate the pain from a sore throat.

Oregano - This oil can be used both in the prevention and treatment of common sicknesses, including colds, certain viruses, and the flu. It can also be used to reduce swelling in the glands and aid in healing cold sores or herpes outbreaks. It has anti-inflammatory properties which assist in these processes. Oregano oil is also said to have antibacterial and anti-viral properties.

Peppermint - While peppermint is already a popular flavor choice for oral hygiene, it has further benefits other than just tasting good. It can lead to a greater feeling of satiety, which can promote dieting efforts, and it also works well in opening up the nasal passages.

Lemongrass - This essential oil is ideal for combatting halitosis (also known as chronic bad breath). It can also be used to stop or calm a herpes outbreak.

Grapefruit - Like its relative, lemon oil, grapefruit oil is also an effective detoxifier. In addition, it offers anti-septic and antibacterial properties.

Frankincense - This oil is best-suited for lessening the impact of mouth trauma, or alleviating pain and swelling after oral surgeries. It can also fight cold and flu symptoms. Just be sure to check with your doctor before completing any kind of oil pulling post-surgery.

Clove - In particular, clove oil maintains gum and mouth health. In addition, it has antibiotic and antiseptic properties.

Myrrh - This essential oil can protect against cold and flu viruses, and can even help ward off symptoms associated with tonsillitis. It, too, has anti-inflammatory, antibiotic, and antiseptic properties.

Coconut oil - Perhaps the most beginner-friendly of all essential oils, coconut oil has a pleasant taste, is extremely effective in fighting tooth decay, and is relatively inexpensive. Also, it can help protect your body against strep throat, a common bacterial infection that can be highly contagious.

Thieves - This oil blend typically incorporates clove, lemon, eucalyptus, rosemary, and cinnamon bark essential oils. While it can be used for countless purposes thanks to its complex blend of ingredients, this combination is a powerful breath freshener and will help to ward off harmful germs.

Tea Tree Oil - This essential oil is another choice that's friendly for beginners. It can reduce soreness in the gums, and will leave your breath feeling nice and fresh. Most users also enjoy the pleasant flavor of this essential oil.

Sesame Oil - Sesame oil is highly effective in removing plaque and fighting the strep throat bacterial infection. It may even whiten teeth, help to prevent diabetes, and boost heart health.

Essential Oils and Health

You probably won't hear about the benefits of oil cleanses within medical journals or other similar publications - that's because pharmaceutical industries simply aren't interested in studying what these powerful substances can do for our bodies. Because essential oils occur naturally, they cannot be patented, thereby offering no incentive for pharmaceutical companies or mainstream healthcare practitioners to recommend or offer them. Yet, countless individuals have experience firsthand health-related success of using essential oils. In many cases, they are able to rely on essential oils for healing properties, instead of over-the-counter or prescription medications that are loaded with potentially harmful ingredients and expose individuals to risky side effects.

Benefits of Essential Oils on Your Overall Health

Essential oil cleanses don't have to be done all the time, but it's a good idea to complete a short-term cleanse if you're feeling sluggish or if you've been exposed to a high amount of pollution, processed foods, or any other type of toxins. Likewise, a long-term cleanse is a great way to regulate your body's systems by flushing out harmful substances and bacteria. Everything from your hormones to your digestive systems can be repaired simply by completing an essential oil cleanse. Essential oil cleanses are especially beneficial in returning the body to its maximum functionality following a sickness or consumption of too much alcohol - just make sure that you've returned to a state of full health and consume plenty of water if you elect to complete a cleanse at that time.

In truth, there are most likely even more benefits to using essential oils other than what we've listed in this guide. If you choose to incorporate oil pulling instead of an essential oil cleanse, you can still experience detoxifying benefits, especially in terms of oral care. The mouth is a part of the body that is typically undervalued when it comes to maintaining overall health and hygiene, yet it's crucial to keep it as clean and healthy as possible to ensure longevity and wellness.

Including Essential Oils in Your Everyday Routine to Boost Health

Though completing an essential oil cleanse or practicing oil pulling from time to time will certainly boost your wellness, like any beneficial practice, it's important to maintain a routine in order to achieve the best possible results. Essential oils are easy to purchase and are all-natural. The beauty of these substances is that they come from the most powerful source of holistic energy available to us: the earth.

While it's not recommended to continually practice an oil detox without giving your body any rest, it's perfectly safe to use essential oils on a regular basis as advised by the brand's instructions. Also, as long as your body is functioning properly and you don't notice any forms of irritation, you can continue to practice cleanses by allowing your body adequate rest in between. That way, your body will maximize its efficiency and stay as toxin-free as possible.

Oil pulling is safe to practice on a daily basis, so after breaking into the routine, it's encouraged to make it a part of your everyday agenda. Practice it as soon as you wake up for best results. Not only will you have the freshest, cleanest mouth that you've ever experienced, but the care you're providing for your body will go deeper and have long-lasting effects on your overall wellness.

More Essential Oils Resources

Essential Oils Guide

More Books by Grace Masters

Essential Oils Guide: Reference for Living Young, Healing, Weight Loss, Recipes & Aromatherapy

Essential Oils Recipe Guide For Health, Wellness & Household Use

Baking Soda Solutions: Cures, Cleaning Uses & Home Remedies

Hydrogen Peroxide Handbook Benefits, Cures & Uses Guide

Healthy Eating Guide for Busy Women: Dieting & Weight Loss Tips

Busy Mom's Guide: Running for Fitness, Weight Loss & Health

More Healthy Lifestyle Books from RAM Internet Media

Decluttering Your Home: Tips for How to Declutter on a Dime

DIY Household Hacks: Organizing, Projects & Cleaning
Recipes for your Home

Made in the USA
Lexington, KY
17 May 2017